SEATED UPPER BODY MASSAGE for ALL

Therapists, Practitioners, Workers, Disabled, Carers & Sportspeople

This book is dedicated to Karen, without whose help and support this book would not have been possible.

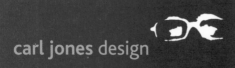
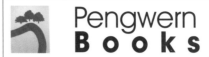
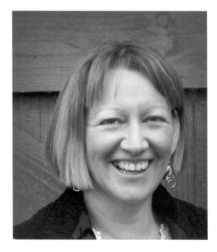

SEATED UPPER BODY MASSAGE for ALL

Therapists, Practitioners, Workers, Disabled, Carers & Sportspeople

BY

ANDREW SCEATS

Pressuredown Therapies

ACKNOWLEDGEMENTS

Following the success of my first complementary book 'Ear Candling and Other Treatments for Ear, Nose and Throat Problems' I decided to write this book about Seated Upper Body Massage. Both these books accompany my courses on these two therapies and are supplemented by my DVDs.

My decision to write this second book came about because I was often asked by my students and the schools organisers who invited me to teach on their premises to produce a book which expands the contents of the workbooks which I provide for them. So if you enjoy the book and find it informative praise me; if you do not like it blame them!!

It is difficult to single out any therapy school owners but I should mention two lovely ladies who have helped me along the way in recent times. Firstly, is Cathy Hamouy who runs the Complementary Therapies Holistic Centre based in Gerrards Cross, Buckinghamshire. Not only do I teach for Cathy but I, and my family, have struck up a great friendship with her and her family who have grown up before our eyes. Cathy is a wonderful teacher and a very experienced holistic therapist. Secondly I have to give great thanks to Sue Bailey at Gateway Workshops in London with whom I work closely and who finds me a great number of my students through her excellent, efficient promotional skills. Anyone wanting to learn how to progress with administration and keep faith with eccentric (sometimes) tutors like me would do better than to study and adopt many of her methods. She too is an excellent holistic therapist.

Two more ladies I have to thank for my interest in shiatsu are Shizuko Yamamoto whose course about Barefoot Shiatsu I thoroughly enjoyed in London many, many years ago. One of her main lessons is that the correct use of body weight and leverage can bring great benefits during a treatment for a client and reduce risks to the health of the therapist. The other person I would like to thank is Sandra Watson my Reiki Master who rekindled my interest in Shiatsu with her course in Iver.

Alan and Margaret Clayton and their family who run the Cartridge World franchise in Wellington, Shropshire were kind enough to let me use their premises for photographs of me doing a treatment. I carry out Seated massage there on a monthly basis and the results have been very good. Their son Sean who runs the PSG company next door must be one of the nicest people I know and he too benefits from a monthly treatment.

Ann Johnson was kind enough to let me use her as a photographic model of someone in a wheelchair receiving a Seated Upper Body massage. She was a very patient model on the catwalk in her home and at my house and I owe her many thanks for generously agreeing to help me.

Guy Hanmer and his family, especially his daughter Alicia and her friend Amelia helped with the photographs at the stables and Adrian Marsh arranged for the photo call at the Pengwern Boat Club, Shrewsbury where Dave Wyatt and Brant Warner were my treatment volunteers. Family friends Rose Bethell and Helen Binnersley were also kind enough to be my photographic models.

My partner, Karen took some of the photographs, was my computer back up, kept me calm and made me lots of drinks during the preparation of the book. Her father Norman also took some of the photographs.

Karen's twin brother Ian Carley was responsible for many of the photographs and coordinating the design and production of the book and he made an excellent job of it with the help of Marcus Clapton. Ian was also partly responsible for the production of my DVD about Seated Upper Body Massage.

The benefits of belonging to a local Shrewsbury BNI business breakfast referral group were apparent in that firstly Gill Griffiths LRPS (who is a fellow member) expertly took the bulk of the book's photographs. Gill also agreed to have a financial input in the book by placing her advert within it. Secondly, Carl Jones and Clare Heighway-Jones of Carl Jones Design (another BNI member) kindly agreed to support the book by placing their advert within it. Susan Caroline who is another BNI member has a wonderful independent bookshop, Pengwern Books, in Shrewsbury and her financial support is an excellent example of the book trade supporting a small publishing house and its author.

FOREWORD

I was born in London in 1949 and studied [up to degree level (Economics)] and lived there until 2002 when I moved to Shrewsbury in Shropshire with my partner Karen and her father Norman. I had a number of jobs in London including being a civil servant and then working as a landscape gardener. Since I have been in Shropshire I have concentrated solely on my complementary therapies; practising, teaching and writing.

When I was younger, I qualified as a hockey coach and played many different sports up to a good standard. Between 1983 and 1999 I organised a number of gymnasiums including a ten year period at a GP surgery, two years at an exclusive racquets club and one year at the Royal Masonic Hospital in London. My home gym which was open to the public had an ethos that led to the social side being almost as important as the fitness training. I found it extremely useful when I was recuperating in 1996 for three months having ruptured an Achilles tendon whilst doing Taekwondo.

My interest in sports and body movement led me to become a qualified ITEC massage therapist in 1987 - my first experience of massage however was when as a ten year old I massaged an aunt's feet when she often visited our house (perhaps the massage was the attraction). Sports massage followed the same year (1987) and then I rested on my laurels until the years 1996 - 2000 when I became qualified in Reflexology, Indian Head massage, Reiki Mastership, On- site Massage (with the Academy of On Site massage), Ear Candling and even mini trampolining.

Having learnt these therapies I seemed to attract others who wanted to learn them from me. To formalise matters I gained a recognised City & Guilds teaching qualification with the support of Buckinghamshire Council for which I shall always be grateful and my teaching career started at the Evreham Education Centre, Iver, Buckinghamshire.

Since I have started teaching my two main one-day courses which are accepted for insurance purposes and have been granted Continuing Professional Development (CPD) status I have taught almost 2,000 students the (Hopi) ear candling therapy and over 700 students Holistic Seated Upper Body Massage. As well as teaching on the day I offer a comprehensive student after care advice service; since the growth of the internet I seem to have gladly offered advice to many people who were not even my students. My courses have been taught all over the UK including Northern Ireland and details of forthcoming ones, and their content, can be found on my website: www.pressuredown.net.

I have also taught other courses such as 'Therapist Friendly Massage', 'Upper Limb and Hand massage' and 'Indian Head Massage' but these have not yet been put forward for accreditation purposes.

I pride myself on trying to be innovative and to this end I invented the cotton Chakra Ear Candling cloths and produced a DVD and book on ear candling and a DVD on Upper Body Seated massage. To complete the set of teaching aids it was obvious that I should produce a book on seated massage.

INTRODUCTION

When I first started teaching my seated massage course I had difficulties knowing what its title should be. There are a number of courses and descriptions for this therapy which is done in an ergonomic massage chair (or desk top massage cradle) and these include; On-site massage, Seated Acupressure massage, upper body massage etc. As a holistic therapist trying to treat Mind, Body and Spirit I thought that I would call my course Holistic Seated Upper Body Massage. This would encompass my hypnotherapy, Reiki and various bodywork therapy training and practice as well as mirroring my general philosophy of balance, love and natural justice.

Having decided on a title I next had to decide what to include in the content of the course. As the treatment is usually very quick I decided to dispense with the lower part of the body (with the rare exception of foot reflexology through socks); there is enough to work on in the upper body to try to improve a client's health.

Having decided on just treating the upper body, the methodical way of approaching a treatment would be divide this area into sections or modules; the back, neck, shoulders, arms, hands, face and scalp. The only part of the front of the body to be massaged would be the soft tissue in the clavicle (collar bone) region which by being treated may help people with rounded shoulders and general shoulder tension.

By teaching the overall massage sequence including the scalp and face, therapists, and others, will be able to offer clients a wider range of treatments and options than if the face and scalp is omitted. A basic framework will enable the therapist to tailor the treatment to meet the client's needs. If a client asks for a certain area to be concentrated on e.g. the back, there will be some disappointment felt, and possibly expressed, if other areas such as the arms are massaged to the same extent as the back in a relatively short treatment session. Many therapist attending courses are already experienced and they may feel constricted by following slavishly a set pattern of movements which are expected of them. A pragmatic tutor will know that most therapists will quite rightly stamp their own personality on a treatment when performing out in the field (literally or metaphorically).

The different Seated Upper Body massage sequences are considered in depth first, and after that there is an expansion of background knowledge surrounding and underlying the treatment and also its marketing.

On my course, the content of which is reflected in this book and on the conjunctive DVD, there are several philosophies/ mantras which are taught both to benefit the client and also the therapist. Both parties are of equal importance. The rules of engagement include;
- Maintain a good therapist posture and use body weight movement
- Good communication between therapist and client
- Work vertically down into the client's body whenever possible
- Only work to a comfortable level for both the therapist and client
- Warm up soft tissue in any area before working with pressure
- Use pressing and vibrational movements which will go deep into the soft tissue on localised and wider areas respectively and will also activate Tsubo points on meridians
- Alternate gentle movements with more vigorous movements
- Use stretching movements on most parts of the client's body
- Ignore movements which may be painful to the therapist or client
- Consider using massage aids to aid, and protect, the therapist and offer variety to the treatment
- Consider sitting down during part of the treatment, this will help prevent fatigue and therapist injury
- Try to keep the sequence(s) simple and add any safe additional movements if this is of benefit to (the therapist) and client
- If there is any pain or discomfort, stop doing that part of the treatment or reduce pressure
- Try to explain what is happening and offer aftercare advice when necessary
- Remember the client should be alert at the end of the treatment to return to work with an alert mind.

The movements contained in each part of the sequence can be repeated more times if benefit is gained (be careful not to overwork the neck) to address a problem. While the routines in the book mainly start with the therapist on the left side of the client it is acceptable for the therapist to start on the right side if so wished.

The movements contained in Seated Upper Body massage can be translated to a conventional couch massage. Many movements which are used on the couch can be used in a chair massage.

All massage, including Seated Upper Body massage, complies with the golden rules of massage; widening, deepening, lengthening, pressure and time. Obviously with specialities such as aromatherapy, essential oils are used and in reflexology reflex points have significance.

On my course, and therefore in this book, the use of the elbow does not form an integral part of the course as I feel that pain can be induced if it is used injudiciously; if a therapist does not do the treatment regularly he/ she will become 'rusty' and bad habits will occur which will be more painful if the elbow, rather than the fingers/ hand/ forearm is used. The elbow can be considered when the basics have been mastered.

If possible, the thumbs are not used for any movement; there are always options to consider such as the use of knuckles. Pain in the thumbs is a common problem with therapists, especially reflexologists.

In the book there is an introduction to acupressure and its history and philosophy. The diagrams of the meridians which are worked on stops at the waist as this is the boundary of this therapy. For further knowledge of this subject reference should be made to the further reading list at the end of the book. Whilst a basic knowledge about acupressure can be passed from the therapist to the client during and after a treatment unless the therapist has specialised in this therapy greater benefit can be derived by considering general acupressure as just an integral part of the treatment and not being more important than classical massage strokes or stretching. To consider a few points (of many) on the meridians is not a full view of the system. Hopefully, the information contained in this book will encourage many readers to further their knowledge of this fascinating and beneficial philosophy and form of treatment.

Most things a therapist should know about Seated massage and its marketing are to be found in the various chapters and conclusions and ideas from this therapy can be applied to other therapies.

The Author is drawn to the importance of stretching as it can benefit a therapist both before and after a treatment session and be invaluable in the prevention and treatment of a chronic or acute injury the client may present with and it is described in depth.

Qualified practitioners can use their specific skills during the overall treatment; Reflexologists can use hand reflexology, Shiatsu practitioners can use acupressure points, Indian Head massage therapists can give additional attention to the face and scalp etc.

The benefits of Seated Upper Body massage mirror those of most other complementary therapies and these include; relaxing the nervous system and helping with stress relief, improving alertness, reducing blood pressure, dispersing toxins, relaxing muscles, improving blood and lymph circulation and working on bodily conditions whether acute (short term) or chronic (over a longer period).

Seated massage can help treat the symptoms of many conditions including; stress, back ache/ arm ache/neck ache, breathing problems, repetitive strain syndrome, eyestrain, headaches and migraines.

The aims and mechanics of the different individual massage strokes are not itemised but there are numerous available good massage theory books which describe the benefits and methods of each type of stroke. The use of the strokes however is seen in the Author's DVD about Seated massage and is fully explained on his Seated Upper Body massage course.

Finally, I hope that all therapists/'doers' and their receivers will obtain good results and pleasure, if not fun, from the simple massage sequences which are described in this book. It would be especially lovely if some carers could be treated in some way by their charges. On the whole, the best things in life are simple and should be made available to all (with a few exceptions).

CONTENTS

Acknowledgements
Foreword
Introduction

The Back Massage
Introduction

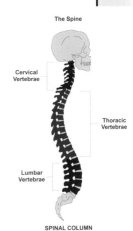

The Spine

The back is probably the most popular part of the body to be treated with massage. Other parts of the body such as the hamstrings or the calves may have to be treated out of necessity in specific instances such as when a sports or leisure injury has been suffered.

There are many ways that the back can be put out of balance or equilibrium and these include acute (short term) or chronic (over a longer period) causes. Also different areas of the back can be affected by different individual or combined processes of change.

Causes of back pain can include;

*   Poor posture e.g. incorrect sitting posture at a work station or when driving

*   Excessive bodyweight for the individual

*   Repeated coughing or breathing problems which may be caused by viral infections, or by being exposed to inhaled smoke in the atmosphere, which may lead to muscles going into spasm.

*   Trauma such as accidents e.g. being thrown to the ground when horse riding or when being involved in a motor vehicle crash. Also general falls and trips. All of these can lead to fracture of vertebrae

*   Incorrect sports techniques such as throwing or lifting heavy objects badly and not warming up and warming down by athletes which may cause strains (suddenly tearing or stretching muscle fibres too far causing pain, swelling, spasm and later bruising)

*   Change in body shape during pregnancy, the birthing process and the carrying of young toddlers over a long period

*   Carrying heavy or inappropriate weights (especially when young person's bodies are developing e.g. carrying heavy rucksacks to school) and using incorrect lifting and stacking techniques - can lead to conditions such as disc prolapse, dislocated spinal facet joint, a sprained ligament or a torn muscle

*   Skeletal damage such as osteoporosis or abnormal curvature of the spine such as kyphosis, lordosis or scoliosis

*   Muscular or nervous imbalances and problems such as sciatica (pain in the buttocks and possibly down the back of the leg into the foot) which may be caused by compression of lumbar spine nerve roots

*   Damage and/ or imbalances in other parts of the body especially the neck, shoulders, pelvis and upper legs (e.g. tight hamstrings) which cause referred pain in different parts of the back

*   Spinal tumours

*   Degeneration such as osteoarthritis which affects the spine

*   Inflammation including ankylosing spondylitis or some types of rheumatoid arthritis where the spinal joints can become inflamed and fused with consequent loss of mobility

*   Infections such as kidney infection or Osteomyelitis (an infection of bone or bone marrow).

Starting The Back Massage

After the client consultation has been completed and all procedures explained, including showing the massage chair or the desk top massage unit and adjusting it so that the client can be sitting comfortably in it, the massage can begin.

The Back Massage Sequence

1. The massage therapist ('therapist') should stand directly behind the receiver ('client') with feet shoulder width's apart, take a couple of deep breaths and gently place one hand on each of the client's shoulders. The therapist should become focussed on the task ahead of trying to improve the client's wellbeing.

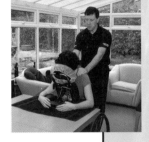

At this point the therapist may inwardly say a few words such as "I want to help this person improve their health". By feeling the therapist's hands on his/ her shoulders in a caring way the client should become more relaxed.

2. The therapist should then begin to warm the muscles of the whole of the back by rubbing vigorously all over it - side to side and top to lower back using the palms or back of the hands in a circular or sweeping action; pressure should be firm but not hard.

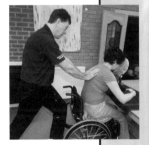

The therapist should position one leg in front of the other and bend the front leg at the knee and keep the back leg straight and move the rear leg backwards as the warming reaches the lower back - thus helping to keep the therapist's back straight in a good posture.

The therapist should move the whole of his/ her body and not remain rigid. The therapist's shoulders should not be tense. Tight muscles will normally respond better to being warmed and stretched with gentle pressure rather than immediately using hard techniques. This philosophy is contained in Taoism (see chapter 9 on acupressure).

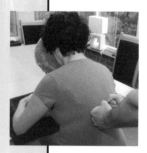

3. Still standing directly behind the client the therapist should press with either fists or heel of both hands down the erector spinae (E.S.)muscle (not on the spine itself) which is the large band of muscle running from the shoulders down to the lower back on each side of the spine.

The therapist's fists or palms should be straight and the pressure should be comfortable for both client and therapist. Each pressing down should be synchronised with the therapist's out breath (if the pressing down is synchronised with the client's out breath the client may build up a resistance tension due to a perceived threat to his/ her body). As this pressing action is carried out, the therapist's front leg should be bent at the knee and the rear leg should be straight; the rear leg should be shuffled backwards so to keep good therapist back posture.

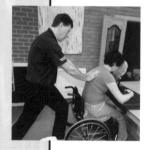

As the therapist moves down toward the Lumbar (L) 5/ iliac crest/ belt line the pressing pressure should be gradually reduced and the mid back/ 'bra line' would be a good indicator as to when pressure is reduced greatly. Below the mid back are all the soft organs which may be vulnerable if excessive pressure is used.

If clicks are heard when pressing down on the E.S. muscle in the upper/ mid thoracic region this indicates that the spine was slightly out of alignment and the noise indicates that the spine is realigned. After the pressing it is probable that tension in the shoulders or neck will have been relieved.

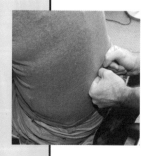

The author always repeats the pressing on the E.S muscle in its upper/ mid thoracic area until no clicks are heard. This pressing is a safe movement as long as the client's front torso is supported by a chest pad or couch and there is no space between the body and the support.

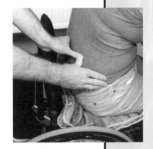

4.   After pressing down on the E.S muscle, the therapist still remains directly behind the client (unless the therapist is short and has to adapt his/ her posture to stand to the side and behind the client) and will press down the inner bladder meridian on the left side of the body. This is done by pressing with left thumb placed on top of right thumb or with the first knuckle of the index finger of the right hand with the therapist's left hand resting as support on the client's left shoulder. The pressing should be done close together in a straight line 2 finger widths (cun) from the spine from shoulder level to 'belt level' with pressure being reduced under the 'bra line'. The therapist's imagination should be employed if a man is being massaged!

The pressing down should be perpendicular so as to connect with the tsubo points, which are vase or pot shaped, which are located just below the skin on all the meridians which relate to the major bodily organs and along which the body's chi energy is flowing. Pressing down on all the meridians, which are covered in all the sequences of this massage, should be perpendicular for this reason.

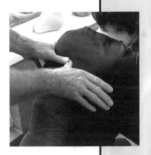

5.   The pressing down pressure is reduced below the mid - back ('bra - line') level to protect the soft organs; it will also synchronise with the therapist's out breath. The pressing points should be close together and not with large distances between them.

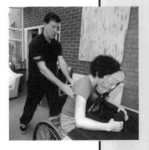

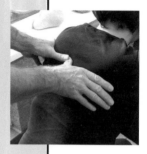

5 Cont. According to ancient oriental medicine the bladder meridian which connects with all the internal organs runs alongside the spine. All the organs' functions can be influenced by treating this meridian. The bladder meridian points are called Yu points where the Ki energy enters the body. The stimulation of the back region energises and harmonises the whole body.

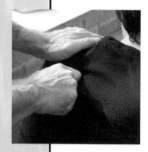

6.   Having pressed down the inner meridian the therapist will now turn his/ her attention to working on the left outer bladder meridian which is located on the inner/ medial edge of the scapula (shoulder blade). If it is difficult to find the definition the therapist can gently grasp the client's left shoulder with his own left hand and pull backwards; the definition should be more pronounced. Pressing down will be similar to that carried out on the inner bladder meridian but with less pressure as it is more sensitive.

This meridian drops vertically from the shoulder level until down to one hand's width above the 'belt line'; at this point it curves outwards (resembling a hockey stick head) to the junction of the back/ side. The pressing points should be the same distance apart as the points on the inner bladder meridian.

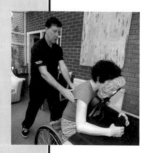

7.   The therapist will now press down on the right inner bladder meridian which is located on the E.S. muscle and is a mirror image of the left bladder meridian. The pressing is identical to that on the left side with the exception that the right thumb is placed on the left thumb or the left index knuckle is used with the therapist's right hand resting on the client's right shoulder.

8.   The therapist will now press down the right outer bladder meridian in an identical manner to working down the left outer bladder meridian remembering to use less pressure than on the right inner bladder meridian. The bladder meridians are important as the excretory meridians so helping to release toxins easily; the client should be advised to think about using the lavatory shortly after the treatment as well as having a drink of water, to help flush out toxins.

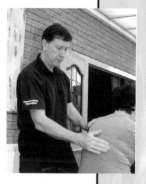

9.   The therapist whilst keeping contact with the client will move and stand to the left side of the client (at right angles to the client's body). The therapist should try to maintain good posture - straight back, bottom and stomach pulled in, shoulders relaxed (if they tense during a treatment just stop for a second take a deep breath and then continue treating), feet shoulder width apart with the knees slightly flexed/ bent in a horse riding or martial arts position.

When the therapist works on the lower back there should be some therapist body movement with the centre of gravity kept low. It is likely that at the end of the working day the therapist's quadriceps at the front upper leg will feel fatigued rather than the therapist's back being strained.

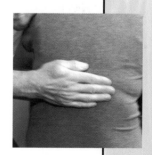

Using his right hand with the left hand resting on the client's left shoulder the therapist will rub his hand (front or back) briskly on the left side of the client's back from top to bottom and returning to the top - reasonable pressure is applied, but as at all times within the client's pain threshold, to further warm up the client's back muscles.

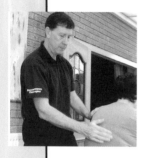

10. Having further warmed the left side of the back (9. above) the therapist will from the upper back (shoulder level) press down with either the heel/ fist/ palm of the right hand from top to lower back and return directly to the top; the therapist's left hand will rest on the client's left shoulder for support. Less pressure should be used over the lower back to protect the soft organs.

11. Having pressed up and down on the left side of the back the therapist will press vertically into the muscle of the back working from adjacent to the spine outwards towards the junction of back/ side of the torso. The therapist's left hand rests on the client's left shoulder for support; the pressing is done with the end of the index/ middle/ fourth fingers or the second knuckle joints of the same fingers of the therapist's right hand.

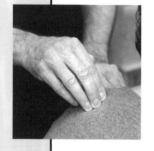

The pressing moves in parallel lines from the top of the back to the lower back (the 'belt line') not missing any part of the back, thereby none of the tsubo points on the meridians will be missed. When pressing into the muscle with the right hand the therapist could gently rock the client's body to and fro; this is a soothing action.

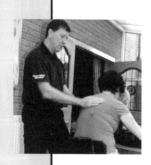

***Remember** when working on either side of the client's body the therapist should adopt a 'horse riding' stance. In the therapist's stance the feet should be approximately shoulder width apart, knees slightly flexed and upper back straight with stomach and bottom pulled in. Breathing should be in time with pressing actions and the shoulders should be relaxed. Slight body movement will help the treatment 'flow'. Don't forget to check with the client that the pressure of the massage is satisfactory; good communication helps improve the whole massage and increase the benefits it brings.*

12. After the therapist reaches the belt line with the fingers/ knuckles pressing, the therapist's right hand jumps back to the client's left shoulder (the therapist's left hand is still resting on the client's left shoulder). The therapist will again press down using the fingers/ knuckles of the right hand but with the addition of a trembling or vibrating action.

Instead of massaging the surface of the muscle a fine and concentrated force enters into the inner layers of the muscle. It is important that the therapist concentrates on sending 'ki' energy deep down into the area being worked on and the hand should remain straight and tense. If the therapist finds it difficult to carry out deep vibration work with the hands and fingers tense and straight a looser form of more shallow vibration can be carried out - this will loosen the muscle at a more superficial level and the vibration will be generated from around the area being worked and not from within the therapist. In addition, this deep tissue vibration will work a large part of the muscle over a larger area than that being directly worked on.

The pressing/ vibrating should move outwards and downwards in parallel lines from next to the spine towards the therapist from the upper to lower back stopping at the 'belt line'.

The therapist should try to maintain good posture - widened stance, straight back, relaxed shoulders and correct breathing pattern. This body position will help in keeping the therapist 'grounded'.

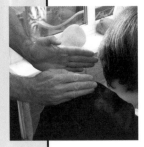

13. After reaching the lower back with the pressing/ vibrating the therapist will apply a number of different Tapotement massage techniques to the left side of the client's back. Pressure, speed and repetition will vary depending on the client's needs and health together with the therapist's ability, experience and fitness. The application of Tapotement techniques can be seen in many movies including the James Bond films when 007 is being treated by massage therapists (normally female!).

Movements can include; tapping, hacking with both hands alternately, double hands 'prayer hands' hacking, cupping, interlocked hands cupping, 'rain drops' movements, pummelling etc. The movements can be done with fingers, palms, clenched fists or forearms or a combination of these. Depending on results gained it may be a good idea for the therapist to vary the routine as this will bring interest to both the client and the therapist. Massage aids can be used.

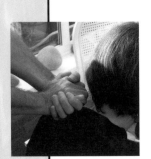

14. After carrying out the tapotement movements on the left side of the back the therapist will move round and stand at the right side of the client (facing the client's body). The therapist should try not to lose contact with the client whilst moving around the client.

Remembering to keep good posture and relaxed breathing and with the right hand resting on the client's right shoulder for support, working with the left hand the therapist will repeat on the right side of the client's back the movements which were done on the left side of the client's back, these are;

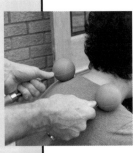

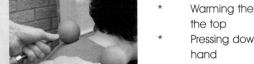

* Warming the back briskly top to bottom and return to the top
* Pressing down the E.S. muscle with the fist/ heel of hand
* Pressing in parallel lines across and down the back
* Pressing and vibrating in parallel lines across and down the back
* Tapotement techniques using both hands or aids

15. After completing work on the right side of the client's back the therapist can then work on the muscles of the whole of the lower back using different techniques such as stroking, frictions and thumb rolls. The therapist can do this either standing or by sitting down directly behind the client. If the client is sitting in a wheelchair with a low back support the therapist may be able to rest an arm on the top of the back rest so reducing fatigue.

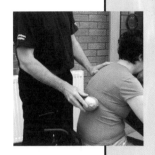

Massage pressure can be varied depending on the client's needs and the therapist's ability and approach. The use of hand held massage aids- whether electrical or wooden can be considered as an option. The use of massage aids can help reduce the strain on the therapist's joints and hands and gives variety to the massage.

The therapist should consider the weight of the massage aid and if there is an integral heat option as part of a machine the client should say if any heat application becomes uncomfortable. A rechargeable battery machine (the therapist should remember to keep it charged up between uses!) is probably preferable to a mains supply connected machine as this will reduce any risks and not need to have an annual PAT test by a certificated electrician.

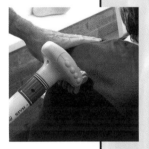

The cost of massage aids can vary from a few pounds to several hundred depending usually on sophistication. All equipment should come with a guarantee and should be hygienically cleaned between clients.

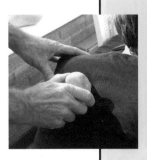

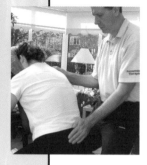

16. After completing the lower back massage the therapist can stand behind and slightly to one side of the client. With one hand resting on either of the client's shoulders the palm of the therapist's other hand should rotate slowly on the client's sacrum two or three times.

17. After completing the sacrum rotations the therapist can stand behind the client who still has his/ her head in the chair or desk top unit face cradle and sweep down quickly and gently two or three times from the top to the bottom of the back. This action will indicate that the back massage is completed and that the therapist is ready to begin work on the neck region of the client's body.

Aftercare for the Back

With back pain, especially if it has unknown causes, the following courses of action can be considered by the sufferer;

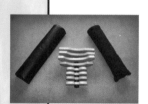

Back support
bolsters+ Flexiback

*   Take appropriate medical advice from a GP or consultant

*   Have treatment, both preventative and curative, from a chartered physiotherapist, osteopath, chiropractor, massage or other appropriate therapist which may include stretching and strengthening programmes

*   Improve posture at work or in leisure situations

*   Reduce bodyweight gradually if so advised

*   Follow correct lifting, stacking and carrying guidelines; also use common sense

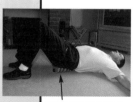

Flexiback in action
to help lower
spinal pain

*   Wear body protective equipment and clothing eg a body belt or corset

*   The back should be kept warm and not open to winds or inclement weather

* Equipment, such as tractor seats, should be maintained properly and not repeatedly used when broken or defective

* Try not to carry young babies and toddlers too much

* Carry ruck sacs and satchels and other bags either on the back or on alternative shoulders if they are slung over the shoulder

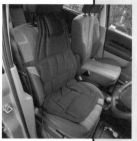

Car Support
Seat Pad

* Young people shouldn't carry out repeated heavy work

* Wear correct sports equipment, use good sports techniques and incorporate good stretching and warm up and warm downs at events and in training; also don't over train to minimise the likelihood of over use injuries

* Try to strengthen the immune system to reduce coughing

* Minimise exposure to smoke, including tobacco smoke, to reduce risk of coughing.

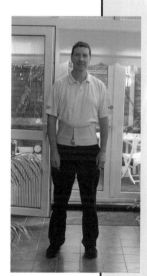

Author wearing
a Support Corset
- Very Smart!

Examples of Tapotement massage movements

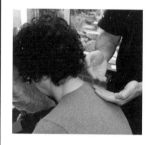 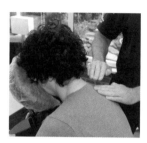 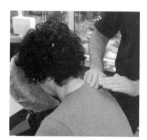

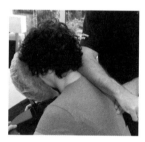 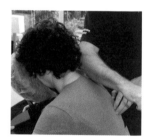

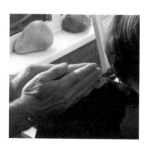 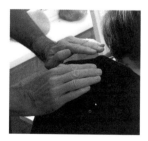

The Neck Massage
Introduction

The neck supports the head and is the link between the head and brain and the body. It contains many vital structures including the spinal cord, trachea (wind pipe), oesophagus, lymph nodes and important blood vessels such as the Carotid artery.

There are seven upper (cervical) vertebrae in the neck and the muscles on the back and side of the neck support and allow movement of the head.

Causes of neck pain include;

*   Degeneration of the joints between the vertebrae due to cervical osteoarthritis

*   A disc prolapse (displacement)

*   The fusion of vertebrae with permanent rigidity due to degenerating ankylosing spondylitis

*   Torticollis (wry neck) when the neck is twisted to one side - caused by either a birth injury to a neck muscle or because there is skin contracture after a burn or other injury

*   Whiplash injury to the neck's soft tissues, ligaments and spinal joints caused by the neck's violent and forcible movement(s) forwards and backwards. The sudden acceleration or deceleration is most common in car collisions and whilst the pain and stiffness may be instant or delayed it can persist into later times

*   The symptoms of a congenital defect such as a cervical rib (a small extra rib in the neck) may not be apparent until middle age when, as well as pain, there can be numbness or pins and needles in the forearm and hand

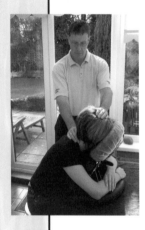

* Enlargement of the neck's lymph nodes normally due to infection, possibly to other causes such as an allergy

* Continual straining of the neck muscles due to bad posture at work or play, poor environmental lighting or the wearing of certain types of spectacles

* Sleeping on an incorrect type of pillow or having pillows too high

* Trauma such as an injury incurred during a sporting encounter

* An imbalance in other parts of the body especially the upper back or shoulders which may refer pain into the neck area.

The Neck Massage Sequence

1. The therapist will have finished off the back massage standing behind the client and the client will be sitting with the head and face down supported by the cradle in either a specially designed ergonomic massage chair or a desk top massage unit.

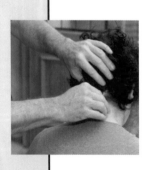

2. The therapist, still keeping contact, will move to the left side of the client and stand at right angles (90°) facing him/her. The therapist should try to stand reasonably close to the client but allow a certain 'energy space' between them.

The therapist's posture should again be straight back, bottom and stomach muscles pulled in and feet shoulder widths apart with knees 'soft' and slightly bent in a horse riding/martial arts position.

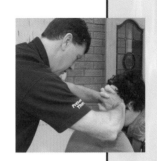

3. The therapist will begin the neck massage by placing the left hand on top/ crown of the client's head and moving the right hand quickly all over the neck to warm up the muscles - gentle pressure is used.

At this point the therapist can consider using a hand massager to relieve pressure on the hands and to lend variety to the massage. If the massager has an integral heated element this may be good to warm the neck in readiness for the following massage sequence.

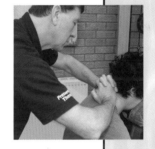

4. The therapist will then stand behind the client, interlock the fingers of both hands and squeeze once with the palms at the same time on three places on the client's neck; on the line of the Occipital muscle, on the mid neck line and thirdly at the C (Cervical vertebra)7 line (the prominent knobbly spinal bone protuberance).

This movement will reduce muscular tension in the upper trapezius, levator scapulae, semispinalis and the splenius.

5. Still with the fingers interlocked, the palm squeezing is repeated on the same three levels on the left and then the right side of the client's neck. Therapists should remember this is a squeezing, not a pinching movement.

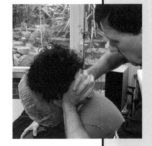

If the therapist finds it easier to do this squeezing movement standing in front of the client rather than behind, it is sensible to take up this position and carry out the movement. The therapist should also try to synchronise the neck squeezes with his/ her own out- breath.

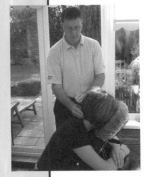

6. The therapist will then return, stand and face the left side of the client and either tap or gently hack all over the neck with either both hands or use the right hand with the left hand resting on top (the crown) of the client's head. This movement will both stimulate the nerve endings and encourage blood flow and act as a relaxing movement after the squeezing action. All through the massage there should be relaxing movements interspersed between more intense movements

7. Remaining in the same position to the left of the client with the left hand on top of the client's head the therapist will by using the right hand press gently vertically down with tips of the index, third and fourth fingers or the knuckles of the same fingers into the muscles of the client's neck at three levels - just under the Occipital ridge, mid neck and C7.

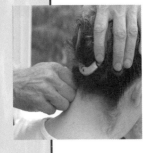

The therapist may find it easier to use knuckles working towards him/ her from a point adjacent to the spine on the client's left side; use of fingers may be easier working away from a point adjacent to the spine on the right side. The spine itself is not touched and the outer boundary to the movement is the junction of the side of the neck and the throat (roughly under the lobe of each ear). This overall movement can be done once or repeated depending on the condition of the neck

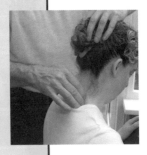

8. Still in the same position the therapist will repeat the pressing movement with the fingers (step 7 above) but add a small vibration to the pressing action. This will have the effect of addressing deeper muscle adhesions and move the neck more as a unit rather than concentrating on more defined specific points. Again this step can be done once or repeated

9. Having completed the finger pressing and then finger pressing with small vibrations the therapist will ask the client to slowly sit upright and bring the face out of a cradle (if one is being used). The therapist will assist the client by placing the left hand on the client's forehead and the right hand on the middle of the upper back and using the hands as a guide.

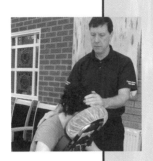

After the client has sat up and become reacquainted with fresh air the therapist should try to ensure that the client's posture is good by helping to straighten the back up with rounded shoulders being minimised. The therapist can then do some gentle kneading on the client's shoulders.

(Safety tip: A desk top massage unit can now be moved away from the client to stop it from falling on him/her)

10. With the client sitting up straight the therapist will stand directly behind the client. The therapist will rest the soft front of the left forearm on the client's left shoulder and gently slide over and grip the client's left ear with the second and third fingers of the right hand. The therapists elbow will point upwards in a 2 o'clock position. The client will be asked to breathe in and on the out- breath the client's neck will be gently and smoothly pulled sideways to the right until a stretch of the neck muscles (particularly the Sternocleidomastoid muscle) is felt by the client (who will communicate this to the therapist).

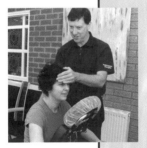

This stretch, like all others in the overall massage sequence extends movement slightly beyond the natural range of motion, is held at this point for about 5 seconds and then the head is moved back to the central neutral position. This movement is only done once. To obtain better isolation of the neck muscles the force of the forearm can be transmitted downwards through the shoulder using the therapist's body weight. No advantage is gained by overstretching the neck or any other individual or group of muscles.

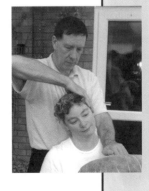

Stretching the neck or any other part of the body is important because it;

*   Improves blood and lymphatic circulation

*   Brings energy channels closer to the surface (see chapter 9 for description of energy meridians or channels)

*   Improves flexibility

*   Eases muscular tension so thereby increasing the range of joint movement

*   Improves breathing by opening the rib cage.

If the therapist is short or the client is wearing a hearing aid the therapist can place one hand on each side of the head above the ears and on the client's out- breath move the head sideways to the right and then hold the head in a sideways stretch position as described above again relaxing the neck after about 5 seconds and bringing the client's head gently back to the central neutral position

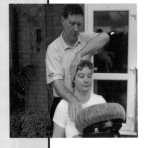

11.   The therapist will repeat the neck side stretching movement on the other side. This time the therapist's right forearm will rest on the client's right shoulder and the therapist's left fingers will be placed over the client's right ear with the neck being smoothly and gently stretched to the left. After the stretch has been felt for a few seconds the head is returned to the central neutral position

12. The therapist still keeping contact with the client will stand as before on the left of the client. The forehead and upper back of the head will be held by the therapist's palms and the client will be requested to rotate the head three times slowly and smoothly in each direction.

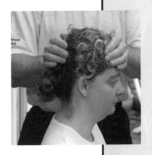

If the client suffers from epilepsy or balance problems this movement and the following movement may be omitted. This movement will maintain or increase cervical flexibility by stretching the upper neck muscles and their attachments at the base of the skull.

13. Still holding the client's head in the same grip the therapist will request the client to breathe in, and on the out-breath nod the head forwards to a comfortable level - this will stretch the muscles at the back of the neck. After a few seconds the client will be asked to breathe in and raise the head smoothly to the neutral position (looking forward). An out-breath will happen as the head is slowly tilted backwards by the client - this backwards movement counter balances the forward movement.

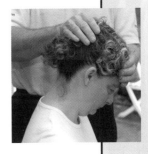

After the head finishes tilting backwards it stays in that position for a few seconds and the client is then asked to breathe in; the therapist will guide the head upwards into the neutral central position as the client breathes out. When the client is back in the neutral position he/ she is asked to breathe in; on the subsequent out-breath the client's head nods forward. The client's forward/neutral/backward movement with synchronised breathing pattern is repeated three times. When this part of the neck massage is completed the therapist will be ready to work on the shoulders.

Aftercare for the Neck

With neck pain, especially if it has unknown causes, the following action can be considered by the sufferer;

*   Take appropriate medical advice from a GP or consultant

*   Have treatment, both preventative and curative, from a chartered physiotherapist, osteopath, chiropractor, massage or other appropriate therapist which may include stretching and strengthening programmes

*   Improve posture at work or in leisure situations

*   Try to sleep with pillow(s) at a different height

*   Wear the correct glasses so that the neck is not strained and make sure lighting levels are appropriate

*   Wear neck protective equipment such as a neck brace

*   The neck should be kept warm and not open to winds or inclement weather

*   Wear correct sports equipment, use good sports techniques and incorporate good stretching and warm up and warm downs at events and in training; also don't over train to minimise the likelihood of over use injuries

*   Stretch and strengthen other parts of the body which are linked to the neck - the shoulders and back

*   Incorporate foods rich in oils - fish, olive oil and nuts into the diet to help combat the effects of arthritis. Use either locally produced or Munuka honey to help with some allergies and to strengthen the immune system. Consult a qualified dietician or nutritionist for detailed dietary advice, check for nut allergies.

The Shoulders Massage

Introduction

The shoulder is a ball-and-socket joint with a wide range of movement. It is made up of the upper part of the humerus (upper arm bone), the scapula (shoulder blade) and the clavicle (collar bone). There is also a bursa which is a fluid filled sac under the acromion (the bony prominence at the outer top part of the scapula).

As well as the shoulder joint itself which is where the head of the humerus fits into the glenoid cavity space under the acromion; the clavicle articulates with the acromion at the acromioclavicular joint. The clavicle also extends across the top of the chest to the sternum (breastbone) to which it is attached at the sternoclavicular joint.

The wide range of movement of the shoulder is facilitated by part of the arm's biceps muscle, the several small rotator cuff muscles, several muscles in the chest wall and the deltoid muscle which is located at the top of the upper arm and shoulder.

Causes of shoulder pain include;

* Dislocation of either the shoulder joint or the acromio-clavicular joint caused by a forward and downward displacement often caused by a fall on to the shoulder or an outstretched hand. A backward dislocation may be caused by a powerful direct blow on the front of the shoulder or by the upper arm being violently twisted such as with an electric shock or a seizure

* Fracture of the clavicle or the humerus

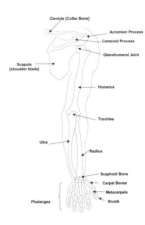

Bones of The Shoulder, Arm and Hand

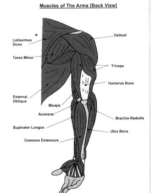

Muscles of The Arms [Back View]

*   Arthritis (inflammation of a joint) or bursitis (inflammation of the bursa)

*   Frozen shoulder (inflammation and thickening of the lining of the capsule in which the joint is contained) with associated restricted movement

*   Tendinitis, where the tendons of the shoulder muscles are inflamed

*   Painful arc syndrome where inflammation of a tendon or bursa around the shoulder joint leads to pain when the arm is raised

*   Constant overstretching of the shoulders at work or leisure

*   Stress.

The Shoulders Massage Sequence

Having finished the neck massage the therapist will continue with the shoulders massage. The client is sitting up for this and the rest of the treatment. Great care should be taken that if the treatment is being carried out in a restricted space that the client does not hurt the arms against furniture or walls;

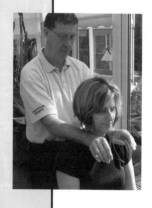

1. The therapist will stand behind the client with feet shoulders width apart and knees slightly bent. The front (soft) side of the forearms will be placed on the client's shoulders and pressed down in three places - junction of neck/ shoulder, mid point and on the acromion point (outside point of the shoulder) in synchronisation with the client's out breaths.

Extra pressure can be gained by the therapist using body weight through dropping the body's centre of gravity by bending the knees in time with the pressing down movements.

2. The therapist will then ask the client to give him/ her the elbows which are bent at 90 degrees in a 'Chicken Wings' position and held close to the client's body. The therapist's hands support the front of the elbows and the client is asked to inhale. On the client's out breath the therapist will smoothly pull the elbows upwards and backwards until the client experiences a stretch feeling at the front of the shoulders. The therapist is told this has occurred and will hold the stretch position for a few seconds to achieve good results and then the shoulders are relaxed. It is important that the client does not drop the head as this will reduce the isolation of the neck and shoulder muscles and the benefit derived from this stretch. If the client has flexible shoulders the therapist can rise on the toes to achieve extra leverage. Another tip with flexible clients or short therapists is to lift the arms back and slightly outwards. If the client is inflexible in either or both shoulders the therapist should take this into consideration when executing this move.

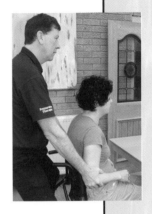

3. The therapist will keep contact with the client and ask the client to interlock the fingers of the hands behind the client's neck. The therapist will turn his/ her body slightly to obtain better resistance and for modesty's sake especially when the therapist is a man. The therapist's palms are open and face the therapist and are anchored against the front of the client's elbows. The client is asked to breathe in, and then on the out-breath the therapist will smoothly pull the client's elbows towards him/her. When the client feels the stretch across the chest and front of the shoulders this will be communicated to the therapist who will stop pulling and hold the stretch position for several seconds. The client's arms will then be relaxed. Again, if a client has flexible shoulders the elbows can be widened as well as pulled backwards. If the client has 'poorly' shoulders with less flexibility the client can place his fingers on the shoulders and the therapist can pull the front of the shoulders in this restricted position

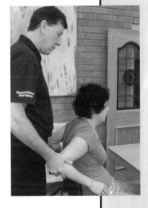

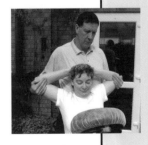

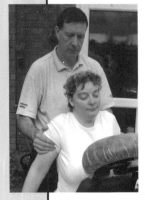

4.   Still keeping contact with the client the therapist will grasp the client's deltoid muscle in each upper arm and perform the 'arm drop' movement. The therapist will ask the client to breathe in and at the same time lift the arms slightly. On the therapist's instruction to 'breathe out' the client will drop the arms vertically towards the floor. This movement is repeated twice more. It is important for the client to drop the arms fast and in a relaxed manner as this will bring maximum benefit from easing tension in the upper shoulders and breaking up any muscle fibre adhesions, If the client has heavy arms and the therapist is slight this movement (and the next) could be omitted.

5.   The therapist is still standing behind the client and will perform the 'ballerina lift' which will balance the 'arm drop' movement as performed previously. The therapist will ask the client to interlock the fingers of both hands and stretch the arms vertically straight above the head. When this has been done the therapist will grasp the client's arms firmly (not roughly) either by the deltoids (upper arms, just below the shoulders) or by the forearms halfway between the elbow and wrist.

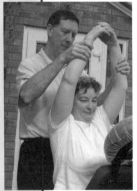

The client will be asked to breathe in and with the out-breathe the therapist will lift the arms slightly; this should stretch the shoulders and upper Trapezius. This movement is repeated twice more. As the effects of stretches vary the therapist should get feed back from the client as to which position of the hand grip results in a more effective stretch.

6.   The therapist will now grasp the client's forearms and by slightly turning his body will brace and support the client's body. The client, who still has the fingers interlocked, will rotate the shoulders three times in each direction. To obtain more mobility in the shoulders the therapist can slightly arch his/ her own back while the client's arms are circling. This movement is called the 'ballerina pirouette'.

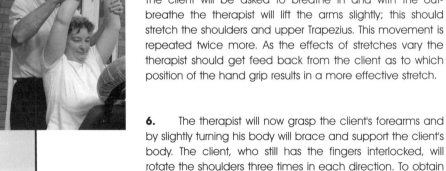

7. The therapist will now adopt a slightly crouched position behind the client with the left hand on the front of the client's left shoulder. At the same time as pulling the client's right shoulder backwards the therapist will press along the line from the bottom end of the client's left scapula and move up to, and slightly over, the left shoulder using a knife edge movement, with either the hypothenar eminence on the little finger side *(therapist's memory note: thenar is the thumb side)* of the hand or with the forearm.

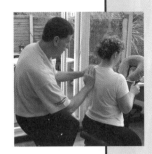

This movement should mobilise the shoulder, work on adhesions associated with the Rhomboid (Major and Minor) muscles and stretch the muscles. This movement can be repeated twice more

8. The therapist will now move to the left side of the client and face him/her. The client will be facing forward. The therapist will hold the client's straight left arm with the right hand just above the wrist (not on the wrist) and ask the client to rotate the arm three times in each direction in a steady manner. The height of the arm will be dependent on the condition of the client's shoulder. A small rotation is better than nothing - quality not quantity! The therapist should try to maintain good posture - straight back, relaxed breathing and shoulders etc as described beforehand.

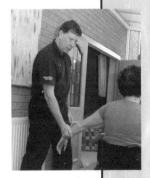

9. Remaining at the client's left side the therapist will continue to hold the client's left arm with his right hand just above the wrist but he should place the fist or palm of his left hand on the client's left shoulder. The client should be asked to breathe in and on the exhale the arm should be stretched slightly and the fist or palm pressed down gently on to the shoulder. When the client next inhales the arm should be flexed (pressed in) slightly. This movement can be repeated twice more.

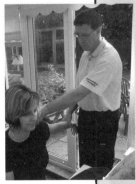

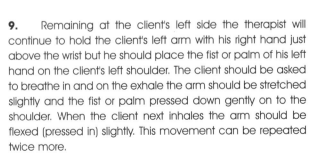

10. The final shoulder movement on the left side will see the therapist standing parallel outside the client. The therapist will hold just above the client's left wrist with his/ her left hand; the therapist's right hand is resting on the client's left shoulder. The therapist will ask the client to breathe in, and on the out-breath both the therapist's and the client's left arm will be straightened with the therapist's right hand pushing down on the client's left shoulder.

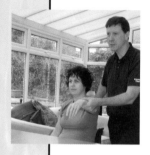

The therapist's outside leg which is bent will flex forward slightly (the inner left leg will remain straight). At the end of the client's out - breath the client's hand will be given a slight tremble by the therapist. This movement can be repeated twice more.

11. The therapist will remain in contact with the client and move from the left to the right of the client and repeat the movements 6 - 9 on the client's right side which were carried out on the client's left side these are 12 - 15 below.

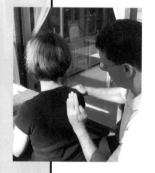

12. Crouch down slightly behind and to the right of the client and as when pulling back on the front of the right shoulder with the right hand simultaneously move up to the scapula using the left forearm or Hypothenar eminence in a knife edge movement from the bottom end of the scapula (shoulder blade) moving upwards and over the shoulder finishing above the client's scapula. This movement can be repeated twice more

13. The therapist will then stand on the right side of the client and face the client. The therapist will support the client's right arm just above the wrist with his/ her right hand and ask the client to rotate the arm three times in each direction. The rotation should be done smoothly and at a gentle pace; the height of the client's arm will depend on the condition of the client' s shoulder.

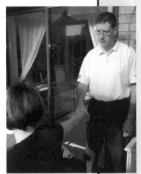

14. The therapist will then continue to support the client's right arm in the same way but will place his/ her left palm or fist on the client's right shoulder. The client will be asked to breathe-in and on the out-breath the therapist will stretch the arm slightly and at the same time press down with the palm/ fist. On the next in-breath the therapist's hand pressure is reduced and the client's arm is slightly flexed. This movement can be repeated twice more.

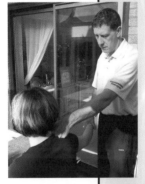

15. The final shoulder movement will see the therapist moving to stand parallel to the client both facing forward. The therapist will place his/ her left hand/ fist on the client's right shoulder with the left hand grasping the client's right arm just above the wrist. The client will be asked to breathe in and on the out breath the therapist will both flex the outer right leg which is already bent (the inner left leg is straight) and straighten out and extend both his and the client's outstretched right arm.

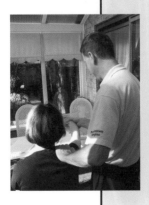

At the end of the stretch the therapist can give a slight tremble to the client's hand. This movement can be repeated twice more.

The therapist is now ready to move on to the arm(s) massage sequence.

Aftercare for the Shoulders

With painful shoulders, especially if it has unknown causes, the following courses of action can be considered by the sufferer;

*   Take appropriate medical advice from a GP or consultant

*   Have treatment, both preventative and curative, from a chartered physiotherapist, osteopath, chiropractor, massage or other appropriate therapist which may include stretching and strengthening programmes

*   Try to reduce stress levels through better time management, a more balanced work/ leisure situation and through relaxation techniques such as yoga

*   Try to correct imbalances in other related parts of the body, especially the back

*   Try to adopt measures which will prevent constant overstretching

*   Wear neck protective equipment such as shoulder pads as used by rugby and other contact sports players

*   Wear correct sports equipment, employ good sports techniques such as correct rugby and martial arts tackling and blocking. Incorporate good stretching and warm up and warm downs at events and in training; also don't over train to minimise the likelihood of overuse injuries

*   Stretch and strengthen other parts of the body which are linked to the neck - the shoulders and back

*   Incorporate foods rich in oils - fish, olive oil and nuts into the diet to help combat the effects of arthritis. Consult a qualified dietician or nutritionist for detailed dietary advice. Be careful of nut allergies

The Arms Massage

Introduction

The arm consists of the shoulder, elbow and wrist joints; the Humerus (upper arm), Radius and Ulna bones. The Biceps and Triceps muscles of the upper arm and the muscles of the lower arm including the common flexors and extensors, Pronator teres, Supinator and the Brachioradialis.

The wrist joint between the arm and hand consists of eight carpal bones arranged in two rows which form the carpus and these both articulate with the ulna and radius forearm bones and the bones of the palm of the hand (metacarpals).

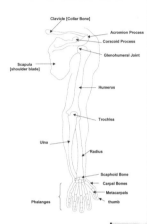

Bones of The Shoulder, Arm and Hand

Causes of arm pain can include;

*   referred pain from neck injuries such as a 'whiplash' reaction to a sudden jolt in a car, or other vehicle, accident

*   broken or fractured bones caused by falls or medical conditions such as poor sight, dizziness or Parkinson's disease. A Colles' fracture occurs when the radius bone (on the thumb side) breaks due to the wrist and hand being displaced backwards - it is the most common type of fracture in people over 40 (due to weakened bones in aging)

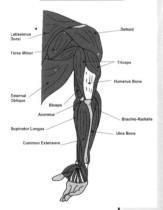

Muscles of The Arms [Back View]

* an overuse injury such as 'tennis elbow' which leads to the painful inflammation of the tendon which attaches the extensor (finger straightening) muscles to the Humerus upper arm bone around the outside of the elbow. Golfer's elbow is caused by the painful inflammation of the tendon which attaches the flexor (finger and wrist bending) muscles to the inside of the elbow; muscles of the forearm can also become painful. While these two elbow conditions can be caused and exacerbated by using incorrect or new sports equipment or changing technique they can also be due to repetitive every day action such as gripping or twisting a screwdriver or paintbrush or gardening. It can be made worse by lifting heavy objects such as pails of water or large tins of paint.

* pain radiating down the left arm can be a symptom of a heart attack (Myocardial infarction)

* a reaction to an inoculation in the arm, donating blood or having blood taken from the arm as part of the process of a blood test

* sleeping or lying awkwardly on the arm or shoulder.

The Arms Massage Sequence

1. The therapist will keep contact with the client and move to the left side of the client and face him/ her. The therapist can either stand or sit in a chair or on a stool to carry out this sequence and that of the hand massage which can immediately follow the arm massage so as to encourage continuity and reduce the movement and effort made by the therapist. As in all parts of the overall massage it is better for the massage to 'flow' rather than be an interrupted process. The client is in the sitting up position facing forward with the arm to be massaged hanging down by the side; the other arm can either hang down by the side or rest as support for the client - adopt the position which is more comfortable for the client.

2. The therapist will rub for about 5 -10 seconds, briskly up and down the whole of the arm - front and back, with the palms of both hands to warm up the muscles of the arm.

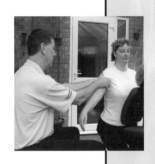

3. The therapist will then encircle the arm (if possible) with the palms of both hands and squeeze from the top of the arm down to the wrist and back up with the right hand; the client's left hand being supported by the therapist's left hand.

4. The therapist will still support the client's hand with the left hand and briskly tap, for 5 - 10 seconds, all parts of the client's arm - front and back, with either the finger tips of the 2nd/ 3rd/ 4th fingers or the bent knuckles of these fingers. The tapping should be firm but not painful vertically into the arm to work on the meridians which are found in the arm. This tapping should be almost non existent over the elbow and wrist joint.

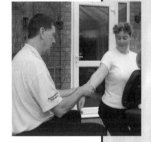

5. After completing the tapping, the therapist can massage the soft tissue directly above and below the elbow joint; the bones of the joint should be avoided. Different movements can be used including circling, pressing and vibrating.

If the client has stiff shoulder and neck it is likely that pain will be referred into the Triceps muscle at the back of the arm. Extra work can be carried out on this muscle which the client may find painful and the therapist should take note of, and act on, any client verbal and body movement feedback.

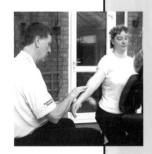

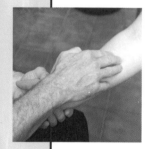

6. The therapist can now work on the flexor muscles of the lower arm between the client's elbow and wrist. Pressure should be directed upwards to take account of blood flow and again different massage movements such as effleurage and vibrations can be carried out.

To reduce the strain on the therapist's hands the forearm or elbow can be employed. To stretch the arm the therapist might like to slide the left thumb up the forearm and slide the right thumb in the opposite direction down the back of the client's hand. A massage aid can be used as well.

7. The therapist will finish the massage sequence on the first arm by again tapping all over the front and back of the arm in a vertical manner with fingertips/ knuckle of the right hand with the left hand, being a support for the arm, in the method previously described in move 4.

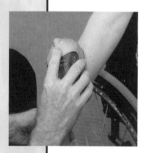

8. At this point the therapist could massage the client's left hand to complete the arm and hand sequence on this side of the body. This hand sequence will described in the next chapter

9. The therapist will repeat the massage movements on the client's right arm which were done on the client's left arm namely;

10. Briskly warming up the whole right arm

11. Squeezing up and down the arm

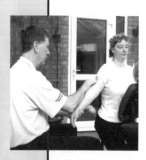

12. Tapping vertically all over the arm using fingertips or knuckles

13.   Massaging the soft tissue musculature around (not on) the elbow

14.   Massaging and stretching the forearm

15.   Tapping all over the arm - front and back with therapist's fingers or knuckles

16.   The therapist is now ready to work on the hands and this will be the next part of the overall massage sequence.

Aftercare for the arms

*   Try to reduce the risk of road traffic accidents which often cause 'whiplash' trauma. Make sure the seat head rest is at the correct height

*   Try to reduce the risk of falls and trips e.g. don't go out on icy pavements, don't trail appliance cables across the floor and ensure rugs can't slip

*   Adopt good technique when playing sports which may have a risk of inflammation to the elbow and use the correct equipment and appropriate grip on racquets

*   Warm up for sports and other strenuous activities

*   Follow the advice of a Chartered Physiotherapist or other appropriate medical practitioner or complementary therapist about exercises designed to strengthen and stretch any part of the arm

* Adopt a good lifestyle e.g. diet and exercise regimes which may reduce the risk of heart attacks

* Tell the doctor or nurse if it is likely to be a difficult task to insert a hypodermic needle when giving an injection or taking blood; there may be a specialist or experienced nurse or doctor available to do the job more efficiently and painlessly

* Try to lie or sleep in a different position to reduce pressure on an arm and/ or shoulder

* Wear protective strapping to protect the elbow or wrist joint.

The Hands Massage

Introduction

The hand is made up of the wrist (which can also be considered the lowest part of the arm), the palm and the phalanges (fingers and thumb). There are eight wrist bones (carpals), five palm bones (metacarpals) and fourteen phalanx bones (3 in each finger and 2 in the thumb).

Hand movements are facilitated by the tendons which attach the forearm muscles to the hand bones. The tendons are surrounded and protected by synovial sheaths which contain fluid that prevents friction. Some movements are controlled by short muscles in the palm.

Sensation and movement are controlled by radial (thumb side), ulnar (little finger side) and median nerves.

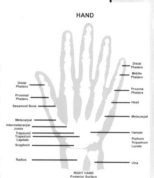

HAND

Distal Phalanx
Middle Phalanx
Proxima Phalanx
Head
Metacarpal
Hamate
Pisiform
Triquetrum
Lunate
Ulna

Distal Phalanx
Proximal Phalanx
Sesamoid Bone
Metacarpal
Intermetacarpal Joints
Trapezoid
Trapezium
Capitate
Scaphoid
Radius

RIGHT HAND
Posterior Surface

Causes of hand pain include;
*   Cuts, burns and bites

*   A skin condition such as dermatitis, eczema, psoriasis or whitlow on a finger

*   Fracture of bones

*   Overuse repetitive conditions e.g. continual keyboard or texting action

*   Contracture of tissues in the palm of the hand - Dupuytren's contracture

*   Osteoarthritis which often affects the base of the thumb

*   Rheumatoid arthritis which causes deformity by attacking the joints at the base of the fingers and by rupturing tendons

*   Carpal tunnel syndrome has symptoms of numbness and tingling as well as pain in the thumb, index and middle fingers and is often worse at night. It is caused by pressure on the median nerve where it passes into the hand through a gap (carpal tunnel) under a ligament at the front of the wrist. This condition is common in several groups including those using keyboards, in pregnancy, women who use oral contraceptives and some sportspeople including rowers and scullers.

The Hand(s) Massage Sequence

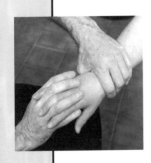

1.   The therapist will start this massage sequence on the left side of the client in the same sitting/ standing position as in the arm massage. The left hand massage will follow on from the arm massage. The client is still sitting up facing forward

2.   The therapist will use both hands to warm up the front and back of the client's left hand by rubbing it briskly for about 5 seconds

3.   The therapist will then rotate the client's hand by either interlocking fingers with the client or by holding the client's hand in his/ her right hand; the therapist's other hand will support the client's arm just above the wrist. This rotation is done three times in each direction in a smooth motion

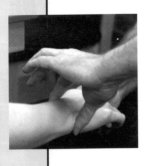

4.   While supporting the client's hand with his own left hand the therapist will gently squeeze on both sides of the client's wrist the small depression between the bones of the arm and the hand.

5. The therapist can flex and extend the client's palm/ wrist by moving the palm downwards and upwards to its fullest extent to a position where a stretch position is reached by the client's hand; this stretch position is held for a few seconds and is done three times in each direction

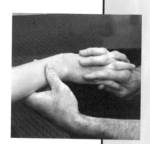

6. Still supporting the client's hand, the therapist will press vertically down on to the back of the client's hand with either fingers, knuckles or palm again for about five seconds

7. Still supporting the client's hand, the therapist will tap all over the back of the hand with fingers/ knuckles or palms for about five seconds

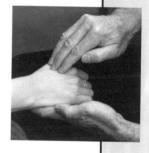

8. Again supporting the client's hand, the therapist will stroke across the back of the client's hand working away in the direction from the client's thumb. The pressure can be firm or light and the speed fast or slow depending on the client's preference or need. This stroking can be done with the therapist's fingers/ thumb/ palm or forearm and last about five seconds

9. The final movement on the back of the client's hand will have the therapist stroking down the hand from the client's wrist down to the end of the fingers or between the web of the fingers and last about five seconds

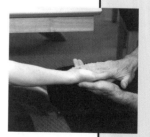

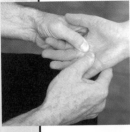

10. The therapist will now turn the client's hand over, support it with the left hand and work for about five seconds with the right hand on the client's palm side, firstly by pressing down into the palm in a similar manner to the pressing on the back of the client's hand (5. above)

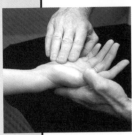

11. The therapist, still supporting the client's hand, will now tap all over the palm for about five seconds in the same way as on the back of the client's hand (6. above)

12. The therapist, still supporting the client's hand, will stroke across the client's hand in the direction away from the client's thumb for about five seconds in a similar method to that done on the back of the hand (7. above)

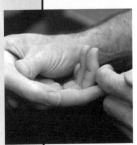

13. The therapist still supporting the client's hand, will stroke down the hand from the wrist to either (i) between the web of the fingers or (ii) down to the end of the fingers and give a little twist below the bottom knuckle joint (first phalangeal joint), which will produce a little 'click' sound (and throw away 'bad energy') - this twisting action should not be done on anyone suffering from arthritis or finger/ thumb joint problems

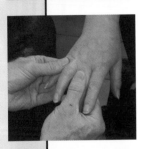

14. To stretch the client's fingers/ thumb further the therapist can rub up the client's palm towards the wrist with one thumb and simultaneously work down the client's finger/ thumb away from the palm with the other thumb

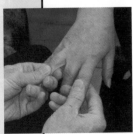

15. The therapist can complete the mobilisation and stretching of the client's fingers by pulling and rotating two alternate fingers in turn, starting with the little finger/middle finger, ring finger/index finger etc moving across the hand and back again – this is the "milking the cow" movement.

16. The therapist will then move round to the client's other side and repeat the same movements on the right hand which can be massaged directly after the right arm is treated. The client's hand will be supported by the therapist's left hand.
The movements which will have the same duration (5 seconds) on this side are;

17. Warming the right hand by rubbing it briskly on both sides at the same time

18. Rotating the hand in each direction

19. Squeezing three times the slight depression on both sides of the wrist between the arm and hand

20. Flexing the palm downwards and upwards

21. Pressing down into the back of the client's hand

22. Tapping vertically into the back of the client's hand

23. Stroking away from the thumb across the back of the client's hand

24. Stroking down from the wrist towards the finger tips or webs between the fingers

25. After turning the hand over, the therapist will press down into the client's palm

26. The therapist will tap all over the client's palm

27. The therapist will stroke across the palm away from the thumb

28. The therapist will stroke down the palm from the wrist towards the fingers and give a rotation below the lowest knuckle joint to get a 'click' (unless there is a contraindication against doing this)

29. The therapist can stretch the thumb/ fingers by moving the thumb up the client's palm and down a digit simultaneously.

30. The therapist will complete the routine by repeating the "milking the cow" movement on this hand.

If a therapist is a qualified reflexologist the hand reflexology points can be pressed and stimulated.

The therapist is now ready to carry out a head and scalp massage with the whole massage sequence completed by a facial massage.

Aftercare for the Hands

* Wear protective gloves at work or leisure to reduce the risk of cuts or burns

* Use insect repellent creams or sprays to minimise the risk of bites

* Minimise exposure to irritating materials such as fibre glass fibres, certain foods, adhesives, elastic, nickel jewellery or plants if these are known to be the cause of a skin allergy

*   Use skin moisturisers, barrier creams or emollients on the hands to prevent them drying out and cracking

*   Have breaks from using keyboards or when texting and ensure that safe working practices are followed such as having a correct wrist support and ergonomic mouse and keyboard with a laptop or PC

*   As well as having medical treatment for arthritis a sufferer should try to reduce movements which will exacerbate the symptoms of the condition and try to see if dietary changes such as eating good quality olive oil or oily fish or having supplements such as Glucosamine sulphate with chondrin will help. The GP or a qualified dietician/ nutritionist should be consulted for advice. A sufferer could also see if losing weight or reducing intake of citrus fruits or tomatoes may help

*   Carpal tunnel syndrome can first be treated by resting the affected hand in a splint at night, if this is unsuccessful drug or surgery options will have to be considered. Good sports technique or keyboard skills are important in reducing the risk of this condition occurring.

The Head and Scalp Massage

Introduction

A massage of the hair (except in bald people) and the scalp which underlies it can either be relaxing or invigorating or both of these. There are a number of disorders which can affect the hair and scalp and whilst some of the symptoms are cosmetic they can be an indication of a more serious problem and these include;

*   Brittle hair with broken ends can either more commonly be a sign of excessive shampooing, combing or blow-drying or unusually a severe mineral or vitamin deficiency or under activity of the thyroid gland (hypothyroidism)

*   Very dry hair often results from the excessive use of heated rollers or perming/ tinting/ bleaching; unusually it can be a sign of malnutrition

*   Inflammation can be caused by ingrown hair's free-growing end penetrating the skin near the hair follicle. It is more usual in black people or in those with curly hair

*   As the muscle sheet (the epicranius) to which the skin of the scalp is only loosely attached to the skull it is easily torn away if hair is caught up in machinery. In the olden days ladies often had their hair (and other body parts) caught in clothes washing mangles. Because the scalp is served with a rich supply of blood vessels, scalp wounds often bleed freely - this can be seen when footballers or boxers accidentally clash heads together

*   Dandruff, hair loss (especially in men), sebaceous
        cysts, psoriasis, fungal infections such as ringworm
        and parasitic infestations such as lice are all
        conditions affecting the hair and scalp. If any of these
        are affecting a client's head the therapist should
        carefully consider the contraindications (except
        dandruff and hair loss) against working on the head.
        As one of the results of a massage is to improve blood
        flow this should be a benefit to those with hair loss

*   Pain in the scalp can be caused by headaches or
        migraines which may be due to referred pain from
        tension in the neck or shoulders.

The Scalp and Head Massage Sequence

The therapist when he/ she has finished the massage of the
client's second hand will move from sitting next to the client
to standing directly behind the client who is facing forward.
With both the scalp and face massage (which follows on
from the scalp massage) the client may derive additional
enjoyment by keeping the eyes closed. If the client has no
hair some of the massage movements may be impossible
to carry out - the therapist can extend other movements to
compensate. If the client has balance problems or suffers
from epilepsy it will be advisable not to shake the head or
move it unduly.

A client should be advised that a scalp massage may
disturb a hair style and if the client is going into a meeting or
having an appointment after the massage it may be
advisable to omit some of the more dramatic movements.

The height of the therapist may mean that some movements
in the head/ scalp and the face massage are difficult to
carry out. If any movement leads to fatigue or bad posture
which may adversely affect the therapist it should be
omitted or modified.

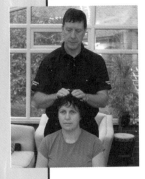

1. The therapist will stroke down one side of the client's head two or three times from the top (the crown) to the nape of the neck with the palm of the hand or the forearm; this movement is repeated on the other side for the same number of times. The hand which is not moving will rest on the crown of the client's head and to prevent the therapist's back twisting the right hand should stroke down the right side of the head and the left hand should stroke down the left side. The therapist should not forget to work down the back of the head. To complete this movement the therapist can stroke down with both palms for the same number of times, working on each side of the head at the same time. To extend the hand movement, the therapist can lengthen the stroking down to the nape and extend across the shoulders

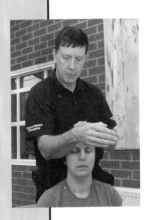

2. The therapist can move the palm/ knuckles/ finger tips/ forearm across the scalp in a motion resembling those of a car's windscreen wiper (the other hand is resting on the top of the client's head). First on one side for about five seconds and then on the other side for the same length of time. After the back of the head is worked, both sides can be worked simultaneously. The therapist again should take care not to twist the back

3. The therapist can press the fingertips of both hands on to the scalp and gently move quickly or slowly the client's scalp, the whole head should be moved, this movement can be called a 'spider legs' movement!

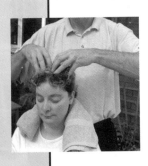

4. The therapist can hook the fingers into the base of the hair and slowly or quickly pull it upwards

5. The therapist can place both hands on the client's head and give the head a very gentle shake

6. The therapist can lightly press down and move the palms of the hands very quickly in opposite directions across the head - the 'Tommy Cooper' movement!

7.   The therapist can carry out a gentle fingertips hacking movement, using light pressure, all over the head

8.   The therapist can fingertips 'scratch' the hair all over the head

9.   The therapist can riffle/ 'spoil' the hair using both hands. If the client does not want the hair unduly disturbed this movement can be omitted

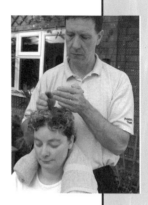

10.   The therapist can 'shampoo' the hair using both hands

11.   The therapist can 'comb' the hair back into shape using both hands

12.   The therapist can place both hands on the head and give three gentle presses with a different location with each press.

Aftercare for the Head and Scalp

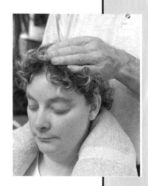

*   Take appropriate advice from a GP or consultant for skin/ hair conditions or headaches and migraines

*   Adopt the correct skin and hair treatment regime using appropriate products; follow the advice of a hairdresser/ stylist or makeup expert

*   Follow a good diet, drink plenty of water and eat regularly - a qualified dietician or nutritionist can advise if necessary

*   Wear correct head and scalp protection to minimise accidents or damage at work, in the home or at leisure

*   Try to minimise the effects of headaches and migraines by having regular eye tests and wearing correct spectacles and contact lenses. Ensure lighting is suitable, maintain good posture and see if there are triggers for migraine attacks and try some of the many available anti-migraine aids to see if they help. Organisations such as the Migraine Trust can offer advice.

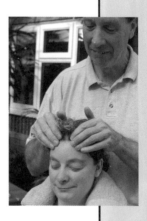

The Facial Massage

Introduction

A facial massage is probably one of the most popular treatments offered to both women, and increasingly men, in beauty salons and health spas throughout the world whether it is part of an overall treatment or as a stand alone treatment. As well as being a stress reducing treatment it is also the method by which creams and oils are introduced into the skin. The main benefits of facial massage as well as stimulating the vascular (blood) and lymphatic systems are to improve cellular activity and skin texture.

Causes of facial pain can include;

* Direct injury including blows or cuts

* Infections, such as sinusitis which is an infection in the air spaces in the facial bones around the eyes and cheeks

* Mumps which causes pain in the cheeks before the onset of swelling in front of or below the ears

* Boils in the nose or the ear may refer pain to the face

* Teeth, gums and jaw problems including decay, abscess or impacted wisdom teeth or jaw dislocation

* Damage or weakness to the facial nerve and this can be associated with neuralgia, Bell's Palsy or shingles (herpes zoster)

* Referred pain can include angina pectoris as experienced with jaw pain; migraine headaches which can be referred to one side of the face; or as a symptom of depression.

The Facial Massage Sequence

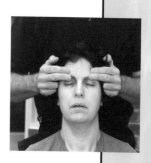

After completing the Scalp and Head Massage the therapist will remain standing behind the client with support to the client's back being given by resting the client's back against the therapist's hip. The client's neck could also be supported by placing a rolled up towel or sternum pad against it between the therapist and the client.

If, because of lack of height, the therapist is unable to perform any of the massage movements they should be omitted or modified for safety sake. The client should be encouraged to keep the eyes shut to enhance the feeling of relaxation.

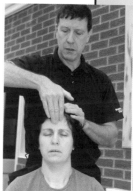

1. The therapist should rotate the client's temples three times in each direction

2. The therapist should press fingertips on to the client's forehead moving upwards from above the eyebrows into the hairline this movement should be done three times and all the forehead should be covered

3. The therapist should stroke three times across the whole of the client's forehead using palms, back of hands or forearms

4. The therapist should stroke up the client's chin and cheeks three times using the palms

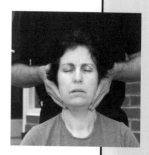

5. The therapist should circle the eyes three times in a clockwise movement, using the fingertips and with little pressure; the movement should be above the eyebrows and not on the eyelids.

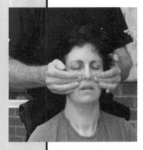

6. The therapist should hook the fingers under the client's cheek bones and slide down from the nose to the ear. This movement should be repeated three time and more pressure used if the client suffers from sinusitis as this is a sinus drainage movement

7. The therapist should continue sinus drainage by using the middle finger of each hand to pressing and holding on the foilowing pressure points for about three seconds each time; (i) under the centre of the nostrils (take care not to press on the teeth), (ii) at the edge of the nostrils, (iii) under the orbit eye socket bone, (iv) on the 'third eye' which is the point in the centre of the forehead about one inch above the nose, (v) slide or pinch along the eyebrows using little finger pressure working from the centre outwards

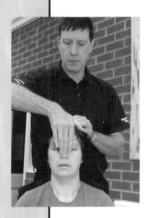

8. To complete the sinus drainage procedure the therapist can carry out the 'salt cellar' movement which is by running one thumb (left or right) up from the tip of the client's nose up his forehead and then simulate throwing spilt salt over the therapist's left or right shoulder. This movement acts to throw any 'bad energy' away from the client. The therapist's inactive hand should be placed on the client's forehead for stability

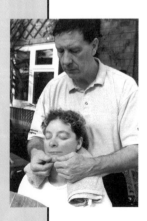

9. The therapist will now squeeze up the jaw bone (mandible) on both sides of the face at the same time from the centre of the chin to the ear using the thumbs and index fingers and gently stroke back down the throat just under the jaw bone using the palms. This movement is done three times

10. The therapist will now petrissage massage on and around each ear including the bony mastoid process which projects behind each ear. To complete the ear massage the therapist can 'flick off' energy from the outer edge of the ear (the concha) using the thumb and third finger

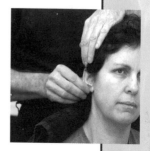

11. The therapist is now ready to complete the massage.

Aftercare for the Face

* Keep the teeth and gums in a good condition by visiting a dentist at regular intervals and following advice given at the dental surgery

* Follow a good lifestyle which should inhibit the effects of free radicals (chemicals) which accumulate and damage skin tissue. Free radicals have many causes and these include; alcohol, drugs, unbalanced diet, cigarette smoke, illness, prolonged stress and over-exposure to sunlight

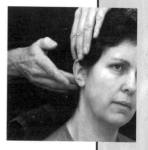

* Wear protective equipment and clothing to reduce the risk of cuts and blows to the face at work and leisure

* If migraines are caused by 'trigger' food or drink such as red wine, chocolate or cheese try to avoid consuming these items.

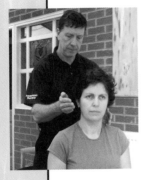

Completing the Massage

After completing the facial massage the whole massage sequence is almost complete. Because most clients will need to go about their activities whether it is at the desk, on the production line or giving a talk at a conference in an alert state of mind the therapist will have to energise them in the final part of the massage.

The 'waking up process' is done as follows;

1. The therapist will remain standing behind the client and begin quickly kneading the client's neck in a firm manner

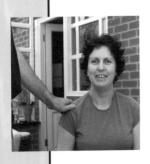

2. The therapist will carry out some vigorous Tapotement movements on the client's shoulders using both hands - hacking, cupping etc

3. The therapist will quickly 'brush down' the client's back from the crown of the head to the belt line three times and quickly 'brush down' the client's arms three times from the shoulders to the wrist. While doing these two movements the therapist should maintain good posture

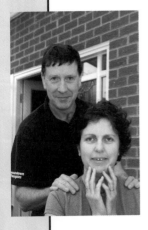

4. The therapist will place his left hand on the client's right shoulder and walk round to stand in front of the client and after a few seconds ask the client to open the eyes and become re-orientated with the surroundings

THE NUTS AND BOLTS OF ACUPRESSURE
Introduction

Acupressure massage is based on oriental healing traditions which are aimed at treating the whole person - mind, body and spirit. It has its roots in the same traditions as acupuncture, moxibustion and oriental herbalism and these can be included in the overall term Traditional Chinese Medicine (TCM).

Probably the best known and widespread form of acupressure massage is Shiatsu (which translates as 'finger pressure') which was developed in Japan from a more ancient form of healing - Anma which was combined with massage and acupuncture theory which was brought in from China.

As well as treating health problems or imbalances Shiatsu (like other types of oriental medicine philosophy and practice) aims to prevent sickness, help with relaxation which counteracts the problems of excessive internal bodily stress and generally conditions the body to reduce any deficiencies in vitality. Shiatsu and most other therapies using similar philosophies aim to make the client whole and it is important that the client heals himself or herself - 'the therapist Directs; the client Act's.'

The treatments seek to point the client in the right direction to complete 'wellness' with complete harmony and balance with nature. Hopefully, the client will take steps in life (exercise, diet, meditation, abstinence etc) to prevent his/ her health from becoming imbalanced with illness or disease following.

There are a number of principles of traditional Eastern Asian medicine, which underpin any of its treatment regimes, and which are interrelated including;

*   The concept of the 'Energy Life Force' (Ki (Japan), Qi/ Chi/ Ch'i (China) and Prana/ Parma (India)) which is found within the body and all around us in the air, water, food and all parts of the environment

*   The principles of the Keiraku meridians (energy channels/ pathways) which run through the body and their Tsubo points on the surface pathway of a Ki channel which can be influenced by pressure or by acupuncture needle insertion

*   The Yin/ Yang principle which is a view on the flow and manifestation of Ki energy and how blockages which affect health can be ascertained and hopefully cleared. Yin/ Yang can also be used to describe and analyse any situation, happening or phenomenon in the wider world

*   The Five Elements (Water, Wood, Fire, Earth and Metal) energetic system which helps a practitioner under - stand the mind, body and spiritual state of the client

*   The importance of correct breathing, posture and the Hara.

Before looking at the above principles of Far Eastern Medicine it may be helpful to look at the history of this form of medicine and how it has evolved up to the modern day.

The History of Acupressure Massage

Chinese medicine developed alongside the ancient philosophy of the Tao (Taoism). Taoists developed the idea of Tao being a 'way' or 'path' into the 'Way of the Universe' which can mean that everything is under the umbrella of Tao and functions as a whole or in its entirety. Most things in nature flow like a river and normally nature is gentle and gradually brings about change without forcing matters.

Massage was first mentioned during the Chinese Han dynasty in the Huang Ti Nei Ching (The Yellow Emperor's Classic of Internal Medicine) which was written about 2500BC during the reign of Emperor Huang Ti.

This Emperor ordered the creation of 36 schools and 881 textual volumes of Chinese medicine. Included in this was anmo massage (anma in Japan). About 2000BC Indian Yoga texts referred to a 'life force' and about 2500 years ago the Greek philosopher Socrates advocated curing someone with an examination of a person's whole condition.

Anmo was obviously practised in China before the Nei Ching was written and while it is not known when it first began some estimates are between five and ten thousand years ago. With such an early foundation anma is the source for other styles of Eastern massage such as Shiatsu and Tuina and Western massage such as Swedish massage.

In China, different ailments due mainly to climate or location gave rise to different treatment regimes. In the North, the cold led to lung problems so moxibustion developed; in the humid South the pressing of the body with instruments led to acupuncture; in the West, herbal remedies were developed from the rich vegetation; the East contributed the use of surgical instruments and in the Central area muscle stretching and massage (including Anmo) thrived.

In the Zhou and Qin dynasties between 1122BC and 207BC regional medical systems were tested and written up and these texts were the foundation of the research which was refined and expanded to become the written texts and schooling which formed the Yellow Emperor's Classic of Internal Medicine. This body of work which was ongoing during the reigns of many Han Dynasty Emperors (221BC to AD264) had almost 900 texts and 37 schools on subjects including acupuncture, herbal medicine, remedial exercises and sexual practices. Only 18 volumes of these world's oldest medical texts exist to this date.

After AD265 the progress in the development of East Asian medicine, and the use and development of therapies such as Anmo was slowed by factors such as internal wars. Whilst Anmo faltered everywhere except in North China; in the South it was re-invented as Tuina. Interestingly, while medicinal advances were stagnating in China therapies such as Anmo and medical philosophies were introduced in Japan by monks who travelled via Korea starting in the 5th century AD.

Between the 8th and 12th centuries there was strong official support for the three disciplines of Anma, acupuncture and moxibustion and degrees in these fields were granted. For the next 400 years there was a decline in the official medical system although the three disciplines were still used by the general population.

In the Edo period (1602 -1868) while there were great advances in Anma and acupuncture there was also a great exposure to Western medical ideas and this cross fertilisation of cultures and ideas led to the three disciplines being brought back to Europe by Dutch physicians who learnt the skills of Japan.

In the middle of the 19th century a Shogun regulation restricted the treatment by Anma to blind practitioners only as a relaxation instead of as a therapy. After the fall of the Shoguns the Japanese government mainly encouraged Western medicine and this replaced traditional medicine. All Anma practitioners became licensed.

After the Second World War Anma and other massage training became available to everyone and in 1964 shiatsu became independent from Anma. About 1910 Shiatsu had come about because many Anma therapists did not meet governmental requirements to be Anma practitioners.

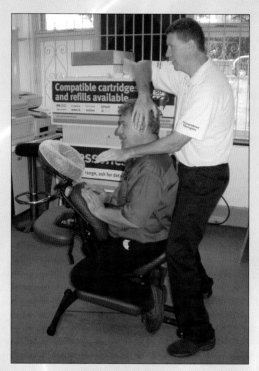

Andrew working at the Cartridge World, Telford Office

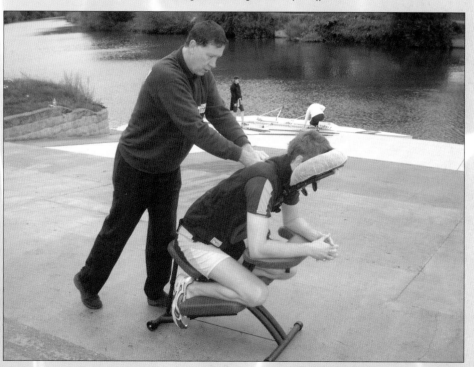

Andrew working on a member of the Pengwern Boat Club, Shrewsbury

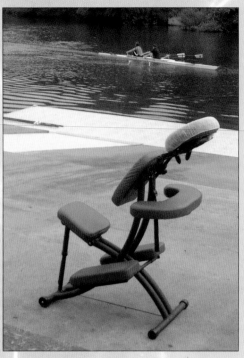

Ergonomic Seated Massage Chair

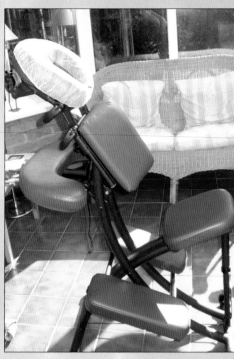

Ergonomic Massage Chair with sternum pad in place

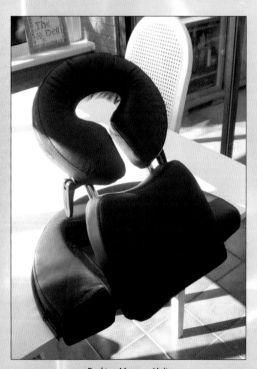

Desktop Massage Unit

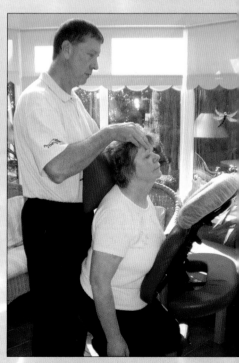

Sternum pad supporting client's neck during face massage

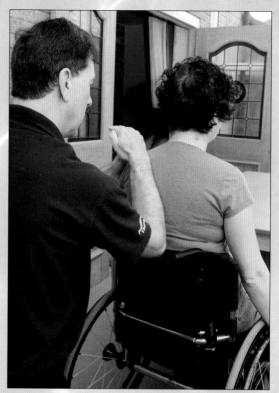

Andrew using a knife edge shoulder massage movement

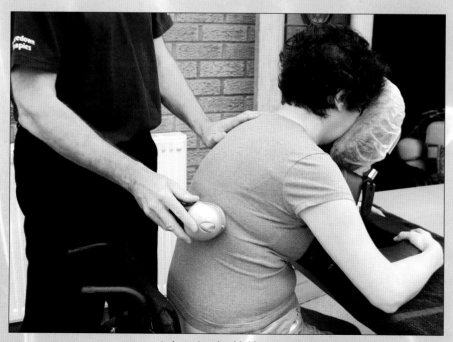

Andrew using a hand-held massager

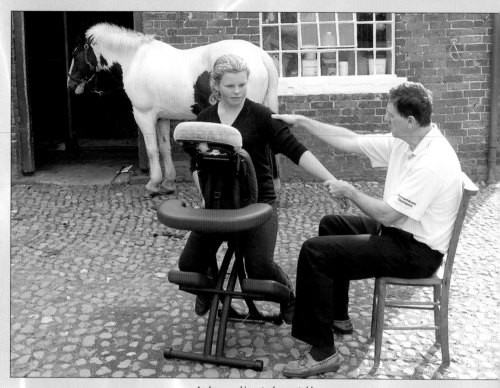

Andrew working at a horse stable

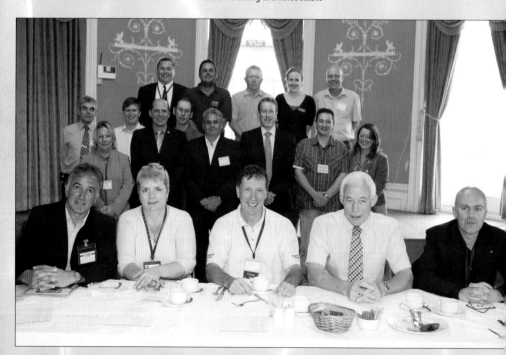

Andrew and fellow members of the BNI Shrewsbury business referral group

It is also thought that they did not want to remain registered as Anma practitioners because of financial taxation considerations.

While there are different schools in Shiatsu, the two most influential innovators are Tokujiro Namikoshi whose system, which is most commonly used, uses systemised patterns of pressure in conjunction with Western anatomy and physiology. Shizuto Masunaga's method on the other hand combines the traditional meridians (Kieraku) and tsubo pressure points into shiatsu.

The concept of the 'Energy Life Force'

For convenience of the reader in this section the Japanese term 'Ki' will be used to describe the term life force of the universe, this word is reflected by the term 'Qi' or 'Chi' ('Ch'i') in China and 'Prana' or 'Parma' in India.

The term life force was included in the Nei Ching book of the Chinese Golden Emperor so it has a long history of almost 5,000 years.

Ki is the energetic power which unifies and animates and by doing so cements everything together so that it exists. Ki is any energy movement within the body such as blood flow or outside the body such as the movement of the sea, clouds, wind or the leaves of trees. Not only does Ki enable everything to exist but more Ki is needed to enable any movement to take place. The more alive someone is the more Ki they will have.

Ki is everywhere in the environment and some places have more than others. Moving water generates more Ki and this can be seen by the activity at waterfalls and when rough waves break on a beach.

To allow us to live and develop we have to have a regular supply of Ki, this is obtained from three sources;
1.   Inherited from parents
2.   From the air and sunlight
3.   From food and drink.

To allow life to progress and develop and change from birth to death another element is needed and this substance is called 'Jing' or' Essence'. If a living entity does not have Jing it is dead.

A third component of the situation leading to consciousness of a living being is known as 'Shen'. The presence of Shen will be the energy allowing the ability of thinking, discriminating and rationalising all of which lead to the development of a personality.

Ki, Jing and Shen are known in traditional medicine as the 'Three Treasures'

There are different types of bodily, internal Ki with different functions and these are;

*   Original Ki comes from the Essence and is the creator of all other forms of Ki as well as being responsible for transforming food into blood. It is found at the Hara below the navel, is linked to the kidneys and is responsible for energy and warmth

*   Food Ki is produced by the stomach and spleen and transforms food into energy. Food Ki, to be utilised, has to rise to the chest and there combine with air to form Air Ki

*   The spleen raises the Food Ki to the chest where helped by the Original Ki Food Ki is turned into blood

*   Gathering Ki (Chest Ki) is formed by Food Ki and Air Ki and is easily used by the body especially the lungs, heart and blood system

*   Gathering Ki is motivated by Original Ki to give True Ki which is governed by the lungs and it controls Ki in its entirety

* True Ki has two types - Nutritive Ki and Defensive Ki. Nutritive Ki circulates in the meridians and blood vessels and nourishes the body. Defensive Ki is shallower and circulates in the space between the muscles and skin and protects the body. Defensive Ki protects the body from outside climatic features such as cold, heat, damp and wind by activating the mechanism of the skin such as opening and closing the pores so regulating the body's temperature. The Defensive Ki is affected by the state of Lung Ki, Kidney Ki the spleen and stomach.

Principles of the Body's internal Meridians (Energy pathways)

There is a network of channels (also known as meridians) which are the routes which Ki energy uses to flow around the body and which connect the Ki to all the major organs and their functions. These channels are different to the blood vessels (veins, arteries and arterioles) which transport blood. However as Ki is the force behind all movement there must be some in the blood vessels and any deficiency of Ki in any area will lead to a deficiency in that area which manifests itself as a problem which needs to be addressed.

Although the meridian channels (Keiraku) cannot be seen, unlike blood vessels and nerves, they exist because they are necessary to be the transporter of Ki energy. While there are theoretical lines of the different meridians they vary slightly in position depending on the harmony or not of different parts of the body. An energy practitioner such as a Shiatsu practitioner needs to bear this in mind and with practice will vary touch to become 'in tune' with a client when successfully carrying out a treatment.

Meridian channels should be in a balanced state. In the Zen Shiatsu system if the channel is depleted, empty or underactive it is Kyo; in excess, hyperactive or full it is Jitsu. To balance up a very Kyo channel it is necessary to treat a very Jitsu channel. All other channels with minor imbalances will equalise themselves.

Emptying Jitsu is called sedation/ dispersal; conversely tonifying is strengthening/ filling a Kyo area. Within the channels themselves some parts are Kyo and others are Jitsu. If the channel is Kyo (empty or depleted) there should be massage before pressure on tsubos; if the channel is jitsu (excess) there is no massage before pressure on tsubos.

As a generality, chronic conditions are kyo and acute conditions are jitsu. Jitsu symptoms are more pronounced than kyo symptoms and include heat, pain or aches.

The Keiraku system has 100 meridians and its connections; it is divided into the kei and raku systems. The kei system has 32 meridians (12 meridians connected from internal organs, 12 branch organs and 8 vessels); the Raku system and its connections comprise the other 68 meridians.

The 12 standard kei meridians are;

1.	Lung meridian (Lu)	Hai Kei	11	tsubos	Yang
2.	Large Intestine m. (LI)	Dai Cho Kei	20	"	Yin
3.	Stomach m. (ST)	I Kei	45	"	Yi
4.	Spleen m. (Sp)	Hi Kei	2	"	Yang
5.	Heart m. (Ht)	Shin Kei	9	"	Yang
6.	Small Intestine m. (SI)	Sho Cho Kei1 9	"	Yin
7.	Bladder m. (BL)	Bo Ko Kei	67	"	Yin
8.	Kidney m. (Ki)	Jin Kei	27	"	Yang
9.	Triple Heater m.	Shin Po Kei	9	"	Yang
10.	Heart Protector m.	San Sho Kei	23	"	Yin
11.	Gall Bladder (GB) m.	Tan Kei	44	"	Yin
12.	Liver (Li) m.	Kan Kei	14	"	Yang

The 12 meridians are connected to each other in the list and form 2 bilateral loops on each side of the body.
In Seated upper body massage the most significant meridians (some in part only - see next chapter) are;

*   three Yin inner arm meridians - Lung, Heart and Heart Protector

*   three Yang posterior arm meridians - Large Intestine, Triple Heater and Small Intestine

*   three Yang trunk meridians which flow downwards - Stomach, Gall Bladder and Bladder (inner and outer lines).

It takes a day for the Ki energy to cycle through all the meridians. During each daily cycle the maximum flow of Ki energy is during the following time in each channel;

*	Lung meridian (m)	3am - 5am
*	Large Intestine m	5am - 7am
*	Stomach m	7am - 9am
*	Spleen m	9am - 11am
*	Heart m	11am - 1pm
*	Small Intestine m	1pm - 3pm
*	Bladder m	3pm -5pm
*	Kidney m	5pm - 7pm
*	Heart Protector m	7pm - 9pm
*	Triple Heater m	9pm - 11pm
*	Gall Bladder m	11pm - 1am
*	Liver m	1am - 3am

Of the 8 vessels which balance the meridians the 2 most commonly treated in the middle down the front and back are the Conception vessel (Nin Myaku: 24 tsubos) and the Governing vessel (Toku Myaku: 28 tsubos). The combination of these 2 vessels and the 12 standard Kei meridians is known as the 'fourteen meridians of the body' which is used for diagnosis and treatment by Far Eastern medical practitioners and therapists. In all there are 361 tsubo points which can be treated although normally not this number are treated during any therapy session.

Zo Fu internal organs

The 12 internal organs are known as Zo Fu in Japanese and they work as a whole.

The Yin organs are dense Zo organs - lungs, heart, kidneys, liver, spleen and heart protector. The Fu organs are hollow Yang organs - small intestine, large intestine, stomach, gall bladder, bladder and triple heater.

Functions of the Zo (Yin) organs

*   **Lungs:** respiration, intake of air Ki and elimination of CO_2 and excess heat of internal organs. Also responsible for circulation of Ki and Defensive Ki (immune system)

*   **Spleen:** transforms food to blood and food Ki, distributes Ki to all organs and is responsible for female reproductive system and houses the mind

*   **Heart:** combines Ku Ki from the lungs and food Ki from the spleen, stomach and small intestine to create primary Ki. Also distributes Blood

*   **Kidneys:** control bodily water, overall balance of Yin and Yang and Sei/ Essence. Also responsible for purifying the Blood and supporting the male reproductive system

*   **Liver:** stores and circulates the Blood and circulates Ki and purifies the Blood

*   **Heart Protector:** protects and supports the heart which is the most important of all organs.

Functions of the Fu (Yang) organs

All the Fu organs support the corresponding Zo (Yin) organs

* **Large Intestine:** stores Ki, separates liquids and solids and eliminates bodily waste

* **Stomach:** breaks down food to become food Ki which is sent to the heart where it becomes Primary Ki

* **Small Intestine:** transforms food to food Ki which is sent to the heart and also helps the bladder separate pure and contaminated fluids

* **Bladder:** transforms Ki, collects waste from other organs and eliminates urine

* **Gall Bladder:** regulates Ki and filters infections from the Blood

* **Triple Burner:** gradual heating in three parts of the trunk - above the diaphragm; between the diaphragm and the navel; and below the navel.

Tsubo points

A practitioner can press, or use acupuncture needling, on specific points called Tsubos along the surface pathway of any Ki meridian where the Ki can be influenced by such activation. They can be thought of as the entrances into a person's energetic body.

These tsubo points can either be fixed (on acupuncture points) or moveable. While acupuncture stimulates the fixed points, which have been known for thousands of years Shiatsu uses both the fixed Tsubo points and those between the fixed points. The fixed points are where normal life processes are relayed to the surface and where there is interchange between the body and the outside world. Non-fixed Tsubos reflect fluctuating functional imbalances. By pressing on the tsubos the practitioner can calm, tonify or disperse energy where necessary.

The tsubo can be visualised as a little pot, jar or vase with its mouth and neck narrower than the base. The neck of the pot is the 'connection' to the Ki within the Channel (the body of the pot). If there is stagnant Ki energy the fingertip opens the tsubo with light pressure; the meridian is entered by using firm pressure on the Tsubo and finally the hopefully rejuvenated tsubo is closed with a final lighter pressure. The pressing, and number of presses, can be synchronised with the client's in and out breaths depending on whether the meridian has to be tonified or sedated. Tsubos are usually located at the nerve ending or between the muscle and bone at a weak point.

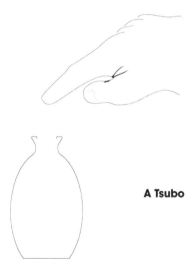

A Tsubo

There are two types of tsubo;

*   361 keiketsu tsubos on each side of the body which are on top of the 12 meridians and 2 vessels - these are the tsubos which are normally treated

*   750 (approximately) kiketsu which are not located on the meridians whose position can vary depending on a person's health.

The Yin and Yang Principle

The development of Traditional Chinese Medicine was linked to the development of Taoism. The Tao means the 'way' or a 'path'. The principles of Yin and Yang are bound up with the foundations of the Tao. They are present in everything and while they are opposites, at the same time are complementary to and interdependent of each other. They are the two sides which both order creation and are the sign of the Tao.

Everything which exists or happens contains a certain amount of Yin and Yang and the amount is always changing dependent of the state at any time; a good example can be the relationship between ice, water and steam - ice in most Yin with steam the most Yang but water is most Yang compared to ice but is Yin compared to steam.

Yin and Yang can always be seen as a relationship between two entities whether it is within the body (meridians), functions or actions. Characteristics of Yin and Yang can include;

Yin	Yang
Shady slope of a mountain	Sunny side of a mountain
Structural	Active
Substantial	Energetic
Affected by Earth's gravity	Radiating down from Heaven
Female	Male
Ovum	Sperm
Lower body	Upper body
Slow	Fast
Colder	Hotter
Softer	Harder
More Wet	More Dry
Space	Time
Darker	Brighter
More Gentle and negative	More Active and positive
Thinner	Thicker
More inactive, slow	Active, fast
Expansion	Contraction
Diffusion	Fusion
More vegetable quality	More Animal quality
Night	Day
Quiet	Loud
Downward	Upward
Water	Fire
Front of body	Back of body
Lower body	Upper body
Internal body	External body

Ki is intertwined with Blood, is its Yang aspect and is responsible for its formation and circulation. Blood in turn provides moisture and nutrition which allows Ki to exist. Ki circulates blood and governs the transformation between blood and the body and demonstrates the relationship between blood and the body.

Yin/ Yang within the body

Chinese medicine has categorised four Yin/ Yang polarities into the 'Eight Principles' and these are the categories which describe bodily imbalance;

1. Interior/ Exterior; the Yin organs are internal and the Yang organs (muscles and skin) are external. The Yang organs protect the Yin organs

2. Hot/ Cold; the Yang functions to warm and transform, the Yin cools, calms and moistens

3. Full/ Empty; Yang nature (Jitsu) is full and associated with excess, a Yin condition (Kyo) is empty and deficient

4. Yin/ Yang Balance; this balance summarises categories 1 to 3. There are three diagnostic categories - Empty Yang; Excess Yang; Empty Yin. (Excess Yin is unusual and only occurs with exposure to extreme cold)

Examples of the Yin/ Yang Balance are;

Empty Yang	Excess Yang	Empty Yin
Sleeps heavily	Cannot sleep	Wakes frequently
Pale face	Red face	Red cheeks
Much clear urine	Scanty dark urine	Scanty, clear urine
Loose stools	Constipated	Dry stools
Cold all the time	Hot all the time	Hot mainly p.m.

Yin/ Yang pairing of Organs and Elements

Yin/ Yang pairs organs and each pair shares a common Element. The Yin (Zang) organs are more solid and they store the 'Precious Substances' - the Essence, Ki, Blood and Body Fluids. The Yang (Fu) organs are 'Hollow Workshop' organs which transport and excrete substances. While each pair of organs is interdependent the most important functions are the Yin/ Zang organs.

Element	Yin/ Zang organ	Yang/ Fu organ
Water	Kidneys	Bladder
Wood	Liver	Gall Bladder
Fire	Heart	Small Intestines
	Heart Governor	Triple Heater
Earth	Spleen	Stomach
Metal	Lungs	Large Intestine

Yang energy is normally upward moving and Yin energy moves downward therefore the upper parts of the body tend to be more Yang and the lower body is more Yin. The Yang energy is responsible for warming and transformation; Yin energy cools, calms and generally moistens the body.

The Five Elements Energetic System

The symbols of Yin and Yang and the associated concept of the balance between opposites is one of the main pillars of the Taoist philosophy which underpins Far Eastern medicine. The other main pillar is the Five Elements Theory where everything in the universe - time, seasons, animals, smells, internal organs etc belongs to one of the following categories; Fire, Earth (soil), Metal, Water and Wood. It is thought that the Yin/ Yang Theory predate the Five Elements Theory.

Five Elements Beginning/ Mutual Position

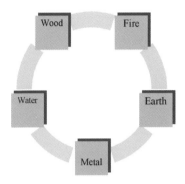

The Five Elements are balanced and harmonious with no one part interfering with another. This would be a perfectly balanced body - mind and body.

Five Elements Creative (Mother- Son) Cycle

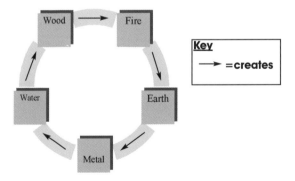

The Creative Cycle indicates the process of creation or regeneration and shows how one element is responsible for creating another e.g. Earth is necessary for Metal and Metal is necessary for Water. This movement can be transposed to tonifying Ki energy, where the creator element is supported to tonify the element to be created.

Five Elements Destructive Cycle

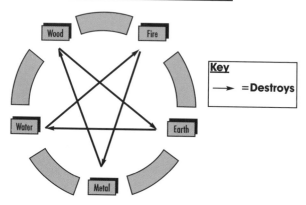

The Destructive Cycle represents the destruction or control of one element over another e.g. Fire destroys Metal or Water destroys Fire. This movement is used for sedating Ki energy. If one element is too strong it can be suppressed by a destroying element.

Relationship between Yin/ Yang and the Five Elements

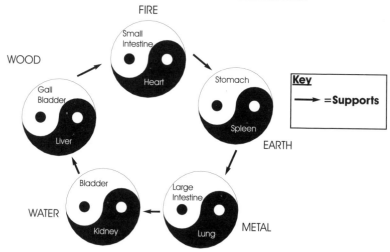

The relationship is often used in Far Eastern Medicine. It is easier to balance Yin/ Yang between each element and then to balance the Five Elements, rather than treating the ten internal organs at the same time.

Emotions and the Five Elements

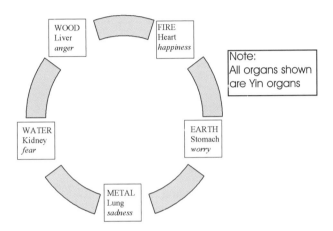

As we have seen, traditional Far Eastern Medicine links the psychological and physical conditions of the body and that the emotions are linked to the condition of the body so any negativity in the internal organs can directly affect the emotions and vice versa.

Emotional problems can be addressed by physically treating the internal organs and meridians by Shiatsu, acupressure etc and any physical problems can be treated by meditation and other cerebral therapies.

The seven emotions are; happiness/ joy, worry, sadness, fear, anger, pensiveness and shock/ fright. If any emotions are unbalanced the Yin organs (lungs, kidneys, liver, heart and spleen) need to be worked.

The Yang organs support the Yin organs. The examples shown in the following table show some of the effects of emotional imbalance (due to excesses of any emotion) on the body;

Emotion	Effect	Condition/ problem
Joy	excess slows Ki	sleeplessness
Worry/ Pensiveness	constricts Ki in spleen & lungs	digestive, breathing
Sadness	depletes Ki in lungs	fatigue, immune system
Fear	Ki descends: drains kidneys/ heats heart	anxiety
Anger	Ki rises: stagnates in liver	headaches, digestive
Shock	Scatters Ki: affects kidneys & heart	strains kidneys

External causes of disease and body imbalance

As well as internal emotional problems there are in addition external climatic and workplace location environmental causes and other extraneous reasons which affect the body and lead to imbalance giving rise to disease or other problems.

The climatic causes are:

* **Dampness**
* **Dryness**
* **Cold**
* **Heat/ Fire**
* **Summer- Heat**
* **Wind (including Wind- Cold and Wind- Heat)**

Each of the different conditions can be interrelated and also give rise to different problems; some of these conditions are outlined below;

* **Dampness:** heavy and constricts Yang flow especially of the spleen. Joint and arthritic problems arise, vaginal discharge and congestion in the lungs with phlegm showing as white or clear mucus

* **Dryness:** attacks the moist Yin and can give dry mouth and throat with dry stools and dark and sparse urine

* **Cold:** stagnates Ki which gives muscle tightness, joint problems and cramp

* **Heat/ Fire:** heat and fire are strong Yang and in excess they can hurt the body's Yin and this can lead to a dry mouth, burning pain, constipation, mental conditions and bleeding

* **Summer- Heat:** again the Yin is hurt by excessive Yang and very hot weather can cause any of the following - sunstroke, unconsciousness, headaches, sweating and little urine

* **Wind:** whether of the Cold or Hot types can cause coughs, sneezes, nasal congestion, mucus (yellow with Wind- Heat or white/ clear with Wind -Cold), sweating, fever sore throats and muscular aching.

Other extraneous causes are;
* **Constitution**
* **Diet**
* **Physical and Mental Exertion**
* **Sexual Activity**
* **Trauma**
* **Poisons, Parasites and other Organisms.**

Constitution: An individual's strength is dependent on the health of the parents especially at the time of conception; the mother's health during gestation and the individual's own strength/ Essence during life.

The individual's Essence can either be drained by an excess of work, toxins or pleasure or be preserved and strengthened by leading a good life with self development processes such as meditation.

Diet: It is important that a diet should be followed which is best for the individual. Whilst generally a healthy diet should include cereals, vegetables, fruit, seeds and nuts with possibly white meat and fish instead of red meat a Yang - deficient person will require more warming foods such as cooked vegetables, ginger and garlic. A Yin- deficient person will need a greater amount of cooling and moistening food such as raw vegetables and fruit.

The spleen and stomach are adversely affected by; overeating food; regularly eating food which is too hot or cold in energy; or by eating food in a hurried way or while at work. The effects of eating inadvisably are shown by symptoms such as abdominal bloating, belching, nausea and 'heartburn' (gastric reflux).

It is thought that excessive consumption of dairy products, sugar and animal fats will increase congestion which causes menstruation and discharge difficulties.

Physical and Mental Exertion: Physical or mental tiredness can often be the cause of health problems. It is necessary to have enough rest to replenish the stores of Ki energy. This is true for both the day to day situation and also for a longer term of months or years.

If not enough rest is achieved, supplies of the Essence have to be used. If this situation continues there will be a depletion of Essence with a lower health threshold. Physical overload strains the spleen because it dominates the muscles and repetitive use of specific muscles may cause localised Ki or Blood stagnation. Acupressure can help move the Ki by helping circulation and toning the muscles.

While irregular and strenuous exercise can harm the Ki, lack of exercise will cause it to stagnate.

The spleen is also significant because it houses Thought so if there is excessive thinking or mental activity it will be weakened. Mental overload will also consume the body's Yin and the stomach and kidneys will become depleted.

Sexual activity: The traditional Eastern view has been that excessive sexual activity will gradually deplete energy. The Kidney- Essence is responsible for the sexual energies of both sexes and this Essence is used in order for ejaculation and orgasm to take place.

If not enough time elapses between sexual activities the reserves of Essence are depleted and there will be an Essence deficiency.

Essence will vary between people depending on their constitutions but it is at its peak in the early 20s. Male sexual activity is more dependent on Essence than female sexual activity so there is a greater loss of Essence during ejaculation than during an orgasm for women.

Women however lose Essence during childbirth so it may become deficient if too many births follow too close together.

The kidneys need to be treated to strengthen the sexual function and replenish any Essence used during the sexual act. Kidney-Yang mobilises the Essence especially in men and its deficiency will lead to impotence and premature ejaculation.

Infertility in women may be caused by a deficiency in Kidney- Essence and Kidney -Yin because these are important for the nourishment of the Uterus.

Trauma: Trauma is a localised stagnation of Ki caused by accidents which cause broken bones or bruising. If the trauma is serious the Blood also stagnates.

There may be a longer term stagnation of Ki and Blood when there may be an external factor such as Dampness which can easily enter the body and lead to complications.

Parasites, Poisons and other Organisms: A parasite is an organism which lives on a host and derives advantage while the host experiences a disadvantage from the situation.

Parasites range from the irritating and socially unacceptable e.g. head lice and fleas through Ringworm fungi to different worms e.g. Hookworms, Flukes presence can be very serious and even life threatening through diseases such as Bilharzia.

Poisons enter the body through different ways including being swallowed, inhaled, absorbed through the skin or injected such as via a snake or insect bite.

Food poisoning is a common form of poisoning where there is incorrect storage or serving of food. The body can also produce its own poisons and these are connected with kidney or liver failure or metabolic disorders.

An example of an unusual external cause was seen when an artist died from being exposed to anthrax spores on animal hides he used to make drums and other artefacts in Scotland (July 2006).

In all the above problems it is unlikely that acupressure can help to any extent. No one should be treated by a therapist if they have a contagious disease.

Correct Posture, breathing and the Hara

For both the therapist and the client to obtain maximum results from a treatment or course of treatments it is important that they both have as healthy and balanced a lifestyle as possible. Obviously as well as adopting a balanced nutritious diet other actions to be adopted should include;

*   Minimising risks in the workplace and at leisure e.g. by having a computer workstation properly set up for the individual or by training correctly for a sporting event or competition so that injuries are not likely to happen.

*   Developing **a system of deep, regular breathing** utilising the lower diaphragm rather than having a shallow method of breathing, not only will this enable more oxygen to be utilised by the body but there should also be a 'centering' or relaxing of the mind which will lead to a feeling of being mentally and emotionally 'grounded'.

Whilst the general centre of the body is the stomach which is also known as the **Tanden (Tan den)**. The energetic centre of the Tanden is the **Hara** which is found just below (2 finger widths & just to the inside) the navel in the abdomen. Many disciplines such as Yoga, Tai- Chi and Qi- Qong and various meditative systems are excellent for strengthening the Hara which should lead to a greater harmony of the wholeness of mind, body and spirit.

Ki can flow like a circulating river from a therapist's Tanden up to the chest, into the client through the sending hand, it circulates through the client's meridians back up through the receiving hand and returns down into the therapist's Tanden.

The significance of breathing can be seen in the alternative translation of the word Ki (or any of its meanings in other languages) which is 'breath'. Deep breathing exercises will not only increase the amount of nutritive oxygen being available for use but nervous tension should decrease. The concept of a receiving and giving hand is also seen in Usui Reiki healing.

*   Developing **good posture** has several advantages and these include - reducing pressure on joints; developing a correct centre of gravity which will allow the Tanden to function better by allowing thoughts to be concentrated on any task in hand (such as when carrying out a therapy treatment) rather than diffusing away; keeping the Hara relaxed which allows better breathing; by decompressing internal organs so allowing them to function naturally and more efficiently. By working with good posture the therapist should be less tired and also reduce the risk of injuries to him/ herself when working with a client.

Developing relaxation will lead to less tension and stress both on the superficial and deep levels within an individual. This will help both physically and emotionally and should help with conditions such as muscle tension conditions, digestive problems, headaches and migraines. Mental conditions such as depression can also be addressed.

Increased relaxation within an individual should also help with their relations with others and the outside environment. Often total relaxation will lead to an individual's intuition being enhanced and this will lead to a 'gut feeling' overriding the intellect - 'the heart will rule the head' and for a therapist this can be an important aid.

The Triple Heater Meridian (Yang)

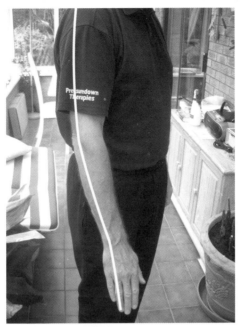

The Heart Meridian (Yin)

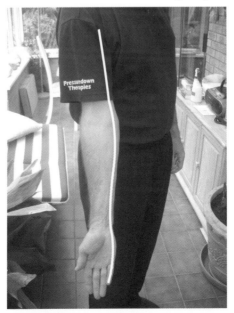

The Gall Bladder Meridian (Yang)

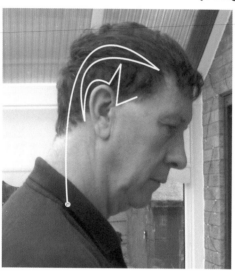

The meridian line as shown in the photograph above is that part of the complete meridian which is activated by acupressure during a Seated Upper Body massage treatment.

GB21 is contraindicated in pregnancy.

The Stomach Meridian (Yang)

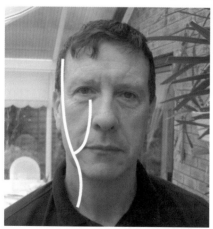

The meridian line as shown in the photograph above is that part of the complete meridian which is activated by acupressure during a Seated Upper Body massage treatment.

The Small Intestine Meridian (Yang)

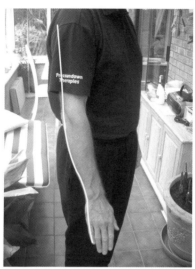

The meridian line as shown in the photograph above is that part of the complete meridian which is activated by acupressure during a Seated Upper Body massage treatment.

The Bladder Meridian (Yang)

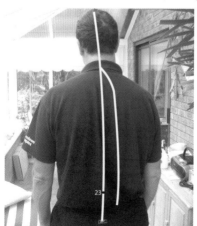

The meridian line as shown in the photograph above is that part of the complete meridian which is activated by acupressure during a Seated Upper Body massage treatment.
Do not stimulate Bl.23 in pregnancy

The Lung Meridian (Yin)

The Large Intestine Meridian (Yang)

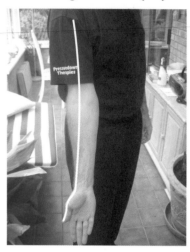

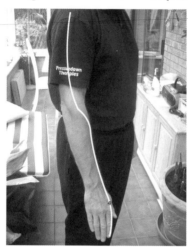

The meridian line as shown in the photograph above is that part of the complete meridian which is activated by acupressure during a Seated Upper Body massage treatment.

The meridian line as shown in the photograph above is that part of the complete meridian which is activated by acupressure during a Seated Upper Body massage treatment.
LI4 is contraindicated in pregnancy

The Heart Constrictor Meridian (Yin)

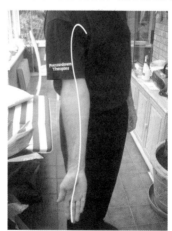

The meridian line as shown in the photograph above is that part of the complete meridian which is activated by acupressure during a Seated Upper Body massage treatment.

Its History and development

Unlike other forms of body massage, which have a worldwide history going back for thousands of years, Seated On-Site or Chair Upper Body massage has only been available, mainly in the workplace, within the past thirty years. It originated as a specific modality in the United States of America and developed first on the West Coast in the computer and electronics area of Silicon Valley, California.

Before the advent of this form of massage using a specially designed ergonomic relatively lightweight massage chair many forms of bodywork incorporated massage treatment. Other therapies had the client/ patient/ receiver positioned in an upright position very often with the bodyweight supported by the therapist. These disciplines included Osteopathy, Chiropractic, Anma, Shiatsu, Massage (in many forms), Rolfing and Feldenkrais.

Some of the earliest proponents and practitioners of seated massage in the United States were Ginger Robinson from Texas, Kathryn Hansom-Spice in Washington D.C, Michael Neal and Jeanne St John from California. The man arguably the most influential in the acceptance and growth of Chair massage in the USA and ultimately worldwide is David Palmer who started out as a massage (later seated massage) therapist but who in 1986 (i) began to train massage therapy graduates in Chair Massage, (ii) introduced the ergonomic massage chair to the world after working on its design with Serge Bouyssou and the Living Earth Crafts Company, California, and (iii) invented the term 'On- Site Massage' to describe the process of massaging clients in a seated position.

There has been an extraordinary explosion in the numbers of Chairs sold between 1986 and now - probably in excess of 275,000 and they are now manufactured by companies all over the world. Therapists now describe the therapy in any numbers of ways but basically the therapist (whose methods allow him/ her to be standing and possibly sitting) is simply treating the client who is in a sitting position.

One of the most exciting developments in the last few years has been the increasing use by therapists of a portable desk top massage unit which fits on to the top of a desk or table. Not only is this type of unit usually cheaper than an ergonomic massage chair but it is more compact and easier for the therapist to transport and set up. It can also be utilised for certain disabled people, mainly in wheelchairs and the blind, who may not be able to sit easily in a massage chair.

Today, if a therapist who already offers another therapy (ies) is able to offer a mobile seated massage service it may be;
*   financially beneficial for the therapist by allowing a wider exposure in the marketplace

*   beneficial to the therapist who may need to use different techniques to minimise work related injuries

*   beneficial to potential clients who may consider having a clothed massage at work or in many other locations, in a relatively short length of time per session when they wouldn't consider having a traditional longer undressed couch massage which necessitates the use of oils or creams.

After having a seated massage treatment it is possible that the client will see the benefits of bodywork and possibly want to experience a couch massage if that is appropriate. Alternatively, if the client enjoys clothed seated massage it is possible that other forms of bodywork which are sampled, as part of the overall treatment, such as reflexology or Indian Head massage may be considered at a future time.

If a nervous or shy client is confronted with the idea of either of these latter treatments at the onset then they may not be tried which would be a great pity.

What is Seated Upper Body Massage?

This is a specific form of massage which is carried out on an individual who is clothed and is in a sitting position, usually in a special ergonomically designed massage chair or desk top massage unit. The length of the massage can be from 5 to 60 minutes duration depending on the requirements, and time constraints, of the client.

Normally however the massage, especially if it is being carried out in the workplace, lasts between 10 and 20 minutes. The areas which can be treated in entirety or in part, depending on time constraints or the client's needs, are;

* **The Back**
* **The Neck**
* **The Shoulders**
* **The Arms and Hands**
* **The Scalp/ Head and Face.**

As well as using many of the usual massage strokes in the Author's massage sequence which is described in depth elsewhere in this book there is an emphasis on stretching and deep tissue work. Obviously the techniques used should be modified to allow for the therapist's technical ability, experience, physique and fitness and the client's reactions to the treatment.

It is possible that the sequence and strokes used for Seated Upper Body Massage can be used for a conventional couch massage with the addition of a massage medium such as oil, cream or powder being applied to the client's body.

What are the roots of Seated Upper Body Massage?

This form of massage is a fusion of different forms of bodywork therapy; some are of ancient origin and others are more recent. This massage combines elements of the following;

* **On -Site Massage**
* **Swedish Massage**
" **Remedial and Sports Massage**
* **Acupressure Massage**
* **Anma**
* **Shiatsu**
* **Indian Head Massage**
* **Reflexology**
* **Ear Candling Massage.**

On- Site Massage

As we have seen, On- Site massage is a term coined by David Palmer in the USA in 1986. It meant that the therapist went to the client(s) at their own location, predominantly a workplace, rather than the client(s) going to the therapist.

Since the early days of this form of massage many other types of venue are being used including; conferences, exhibitions, shopping centres, sports events and airports. The author saw a room full of seated massage chairs at Bangkok airport recently filled with passengers gratefully receiving their treatment from busy therapists.

There is a specific 10 to 20 minutes sequence which is known as a Kata and the therapist works on a seated client who is fully clothed. The massage concentrates on acupressure and meridians and these are common to Shiatsu and Anma which are Japanese therapies.

Swedish massage

Although the history of massage can be traced back at least 5,000 years to the Chinese it is to a Swede, Professor Per Henrik Ling (1776 - 1839) that we are indebted for the modern concept of massage based on the body's anatomy and physiology. In the 19th century he codified the movements, such as Effleurage; Petrissage; Kneading and Tapotement and their results, which are still used in many of today's massage sessions.

Normally Swedish massage is carried out on a massage couch (plinth) with the client wearing underwear; with the body (except the part being worked on) being discreetly covered with a towel or sheet. The therapist will normally use some form of massage medium - oil, cream or powder - to help the different massage strokes 'flow' over the client's body. A treatment can take up to 90 minutes.

If the client is only having part of the body treated e.g. back and shoulders, the treatment will be shorter. If an aromatherapy massage is being done the aromatherapist will add specific essential oils to a carrier/ base oil to target a specific physical or emotional problem the client may have.

Some Swedish massage therapists will use massage equipment and massage tools if applicable to reduce the strain on their own bodies and to vary a treatment session. Clients should be given after care advice on lifestyle, stretching, exercise and diet as part of the overall treatment.

The classical Swedish massage strokes are Effleurage, Petrissage, Kneading, Tapotement, Cupping, Hacking, Vibrations and Frictions. These strokes have different purposes so while Effleurage for example can be used mainly for relaxation and linking movements, Tapotement can be used for stimulation. Kneading will break down fatty tissue and eliminate waste products from deep tissue and Vibrations can loosen scar tissue. There are different purposes and methods of applying the different strokes and there are many reputable massage courses and excellent text books dealing with the subject.

Remedial and Sports Massage

While Swedish massage is the basis of most Western types of massage there tends to be the misconception that sports and remedial massage is only aimed at the injured sportsperson and that remedial massage is only used on people recovering from an operation. It is the author's view that many of the specialised techniques employed in remedial and sports massage are applicable to all people who suffer an acute injury or chronic condition whether due to sports or in everyday life. Having suffered a ruptured Achilles tendon while doing the martial art Taekwondo he was surprised when his surgeon told him that the most common cause of this injury was when people slipped off the edge of a pavement kerb or in the shower. 'Tennis elbow' or 'Golfer's elbow', which are due to a long term build up of tension around the elbow joint due to repetitive gripping, are as likely to affect those who have digging as part of their job or leisure activity as those who play the two specific sports whose names are synonymous with the conditions.

Sports massage therapists often work in changing rooms, at trackside and on sports courts. Professional tennis players have physical therapists available at all tournaments and they often treat players on court. Sports massage therapists make great use of aids such as ice and machinery such as ultrasound, TENS and interferential. They also advocate regular massage as a preventative to injury and to assist recovery after an operation - the Author once took a mature lady client to a hospital gymnasium twice a week for three months before a hip replacement operation, with a gradual increase in daily walking after the operation (which was very successful); the lady did not need to use a walking stick after three weeks which was very satisfying for all concerned - client, surgeon and therapist! The sports massage therapist should offer suitable advice to clients in a similar vein to that given by Swedish massage therapists. A treatment will vary in duration depending on the injury or condition being treated.

Acupressure Massage

Acupressure massage is based on oriental healing traditions which are aimed at treating the 'whole' person - Mind, body and Spirit. It has its roots in the same traditions as acupuncture (which uses special needles), moxibustion, oriental herbalism and these can be included in the overall term Traditional Chinese Medicine (TCM).

The therapist will treat the client in a way that encourages him/ her to understand that the mind or body has become unbalanced and this has led to a health problem developing. Following this acceptance the client will be advised to take steps in life - diet, lifestyle, abstinence etc which will try to recover health equilibrium.

There are a number of principles which the acupressure therapist tries to incorporate into the treatment and these include;

*   The concept of the life energy force, Ki (or its equivalent)

*   The principles of meridian energy pathways which run through the body and the Tsubo points on the meridians which can be activated by pressure

*   The Yin and Yang principle of balance within the order of life both within the body and in all other things in the world

*   The Five Elements energetic system which indicates the state of the client's overall health

*   The importance of correct breathing and the effect it has on the client and the efficiency of the therapist.

The most common forms of acupressure are Shiatsu and Anma and these can be done with the client lying on a futon on the floor where the therapist and client are most 'grounded' or with the client lying on a massage couch.

If the client does take off any clothes when having a couch massage the body should be discreetly covered. During a treatment the client may be in a sitting position with the therapist supporting the bodyweight. No massage medium is used and as well as pressing, kneading and vibrating on specific acupressure points and areas there is a large amount of stretching and vibrating of the body.

A very specific branch of acupressure is Auricular therapy whereby the different parts of the outer ear flap (Auricle/ Pinna) correspond to the various parts of the body and its systems. As well as massaging the different parts of the auricle to stimulate the points small magnets and seeds are temporarily attached to the points to give longer stimulation between treatments.

Auricular therapy can be successful in detoxing addicts and helping with cravings - it is available in some prisons in the UK to help inmates on treatment programmes.

An example of the success of acupressure massage in treating chronic low back pain in 129 volunteers in Taiwan in a controlled trial in 2004 was reported in the British Medical Journal (London) BMJ 2006;332:696-700 (25 March) when the conclusion was that acupressure was effective in reducing low back pain in terms of pain scores, functional status and disability. The effect was not only seen in the short term but lasted for six months.

Anma

Anma is a specific acupressure therapy which while associated with Japan actually started as Anmo in central China and was taken to Japan in the 5th century by monks who travelled via Korea. Whilst Anma flourished generally in Japan in the 19th century the Shoguns limited Anma practitioners to blind people and after the fall of the Shoguns all Anma practitioners had to be licensed. Anma was the basis of Shiatsu which is another specific acupressure massage therapy.

Anma practitioners follow the principles of Traditional Eastern medicine as listed earlier; during a treatment which lasts up to 90 minutes they use kneading, percussion, vibration and other massage techniques. After care advice will also be given.

Shiatsu

Shiatsu is another Japanese acupressure therapy and it developed from Anma. Founded around 1910 it came about because many Anma practitioners did not meet prevailing governmental requirements, there were also financial requirements to be considered. In 1964 Shiatsu became independent from Anma.

There are different schools in Shiatsu and the two most influential innovators are Tokujiro Namikoshi whose system is most commonly used employs systemised pressure patterns together with Western anatomy and physiology. Shizuto Masunaga however combines traditional meridians and Tsubo pressure points into shiatsu.

Shiatsu is based on pressure techniques and does not use kneading or percussion although it does utilise vibration techniques. A session normally lasts one hour and the client remains clothed. Neither Shiatsu nor Anma practitioners use lubricants.

Indian Head Massage

This gentle therapy system evolved in India over a thousand years ago. While it originally only addressed the head and hair, in modern times it has been extended to cover the upper back, neck, shoulders, upper arms, scalp, hair and the face. It therefore has a long history and its techniques and their meaning were often passed from mother to daughter.

The techniques were adopted and adapted by barbers who included a head massage as part of the haircut process. Perhaps one of the most significant figures in bringing this therapy into the United Kingdom in the past thirty years has been Narendra Mehta, who with his wife Kundan, has been instrumental in writing about, demonstrating and teaching this therapy.

Indian Head Massage is not only beneficial in helping hair growth (by stimulating blood flow to the follicles with an increased supply of nutrients) but it also provides relief from aches and pains and helps combat stress. It works on the physical and emotional levels to hopefully improve stiff necks and shoulders, eyestrain, headaches and migraines.

Massage was part of the Ayurvedic medical system which goes back almost 4,000 years. This system aims to balance the health of the individual and within this system there is a balancing of the 7 chakra energy centres within the body especially the three higher charkas - the Crown chakra (Sahasrara), the Third Eye chakra (Ajna) and the Throat charka (Vishuddha).

In a traditional Indian Head Massage, different oils such as coconut, almond, sesame, mustard and henna are used at different times of the year and for different therapeutic reasons.

Reflexology

This is an ancient therapy first recorded in ancient Egypt 2330BC) but probably also known in ancient India and China. It has been developed in the last hundred years mainly by the Americans such as Dr William H Fitzgerald who developed the body zone therapy (a forerunner to modern reflexology), Dr Shelby Riley and Eunice Ingham. Prominent modern reflexologists include Anthony Porter, Beryl Crane, Doreen Bayly, Nicola Hall and Dwight D Byers.

Eunice Ingham found that different points on the feet or hands corresponded to different parts of the body or its organs or systems and they are linked by energy lines. By working on these reflex points disequilibrium which exists in the body caused by blockages in these energy lines can be reduced and bodily function improved. A treatment session will last for up to one hour and cream, powder or oil is applied to the feet or hands to assist the therapist. In a Seated massage treatment a qualified reflexologist can work the hand reflex points when the hands are being treated.

Ear Candling Massage

A massage is a part of the treatment which follows the completion of the burning of the special ear candles. The massage is to the face and neck and is aimed at improving blood and lymphatic circulation, addressing sinusitis and rhinitis, assisting relaxation and sleep problems, stimulating reflex zones, palpating the TMJ jaw joint, toning muscles and completing the treatment in an holistic manner amongst other reasons.

During a Seated massage treatment many of the ear candling face and neck massage techniques can be employed and the ear auricle massage techniques are similar to those used in auricular (ear) acupressure massage therapy. The face and neck massage part of an overall ear candling session should take between 15 and 20 minutes.

Where can the Seated Upper Body massage be carried out?

Because there is no need for a conventional massage couch (plinth) to be set up and with a client merely sitting usually in a massage chair or using a desk top massage unit this type of massage can be carried out in most types of location.

It is preferable for the venue to be a private space as this may reassure the client that nothing said in confidence to the therapist will be overheard by a third party also that no-one else will interfere or accidentally knock the massage chair or the client who may be sitting on it. Often the session will be carried out in an open space such as in the atrium of a shopping centre, in an open plan office at the desk of the client e.g. in a dealing room in the City of London or at a telephone call centre where the client has to remain at the workstation to either watch a computer screen or answer important incoming phone calls.

The area in which the treatment sessions are to be carried out should be large enough to accommodate the therapist, client and a massage chair without any risk to either party through lack of space when massage movements are being carried out e.g. when the therapist stretches the client's arms out sideways and rotates them or when the therapist moves his/ her straight leg backwards when pressing on the client's back.

There should be room for the clients to hang up any jackets, ties or jumpers which are taken off and for any valuables such as mobile phones, wallets and keys which may be removed from the trouser pockets and eye glasses and jewellery which may be taken off and placed in a receptacle. The client should know that any items removed are in the view of the therapist - anything placed behind, and out of sight of, the therapist may be a temptation for an opportunist thief who may be passing.

It is better for the environment to be as conducive for the treatment as possible for both the therapist and the client(s). If there is a window to the room which can be opened this will raise the spirits of the therapist and bring in (hopefully) fresh air. Many rooms in offices and shops have individual air conditioning and heating controls and the room's temperature should be adjusted so that it is comfortable for both parties. In a hot spell if there is no air conditioning a fan should be used and a small hot air fan assisted blower might be needed if the heating fails.

Before using a room for the first time it is advisable for the therapist to inspect the space to get a 'feel for the place' and should any controls be explained by the person responsible for introducing the therapist into the working environment.

There should also be a table where the therapist can keep any items such as massage tools and paperwork - brochures, consultation forms etc and two chairs for use if the client needs to be asked any questions either before or after the treatment. A bonus is accessibility to a fresh drinking water source, a kitchen or even the staff canteen for lunch. If the massage room can be locked this will mean the massage chair and any other items can be kept safely when the therapist is away from the room at any time.

It is important for the therapist to know the location of the nearest toilet and the fire escape and any fire regulations and procedures (such as when the regular fire drills take place).

In an office location it may be irritating for other members of staff in the surrounding vicinity to be exposed to music or other accompanying sound. In other locations such as in a sports changing facility music may be well received by competitors. It is often important to keep the sound of the conversation between the client and therapist to a minimum. If no music is played that will be one less item for the therapist to remember (or forget) to take to the venue.

Possible seated massage venues include;

* **The office, factory, production facility or showroom**

* **In the home**

* **Exhibitions and trade shows (for visitors and staff manning the stands) including product launches and student employment fairs**

* **Shopping malls and department stores**

* **Conferences, conventions and workshops**

* **Athletics and other sports events - for contestants, support staff and spectators**

* **Airports, ferry ports and onboard ships and aircraft**

* **Tourist locations such as the beach or on the promenade**

* **Health spas and hair salons**

* **Residents' common lounges in retirement flats and nursing homes**

* **Hospitals, clinics and dental practices**

* **Archaeology sites**

* **Fetes and fairs**

* **Music and Culture festivals**

* **Parties and banquets.**

How long should the Seated Upper Body massage take?

In the workplace it is unlikely that the client will have more than 20 minutes available for a treatment. This duration will include any consultation and the minor adjustment of outer clothing.

A specific massage sequence, or Kata, can be varied to take account of;

* **Physical or emotional conditions and needs the client may have**

* **Time constraints on the massage**

* **Experience or skills of the therapist**

* **Physical capabilities of the therapist.**

The therapist can both shorten the massage duration but conversely can lengthen it if necessary. It may be that a company CEO needs a longer time than someone who is more junior; the junior may however be given a longer time as a reward for pulling off a good deal for the company.

The length of time for each massage must be decided in consultation with the representative of the company or organisation where the therapist is working. An advantage of Seated Upper Body massage is that its sequence and techniques can be easily adapted to a conventional massage couch treatment and carried out over a longer period simply by multiplying the number of each stroke.

In the sporting context the seated massage can be carried out both before and after the event. A therapist should ensure that protective covers are used on any equipment if the client(s) is sweaty, muddy or wet after a sports event! At a production facility similar protective precautions may need to be taken - the author once worked for a week at a confectionery factory and the workers were not allowed to remove hygienic over - boots or their overalls which were caked in sugar.

Who benefits from Seated Upper Body massage?

There are several main groups who benefit from this specific form of massage and the main ones;

*   have a limited amount of available time; a seated massage can take much less time than a traditional couch massage

*   need to have the therapist come to the client's location

*   do not like the application of any type of massage medium - oil, cream or powder. There may be the worry about an allergic reaction or the risk of ruining clothing

*   do not want to remove much clothing whether for religious reasons or may be shy of their body's appearance to another person (the therapist)

*   suffer from upper body physical problems such as back pain, stiff shoulders, stress related headaches or certain emotional situations which may be helped by communicating with an independent person (the therapist)

*   find it difficult to sleep - many clients can, and need to, go to sleep during the bulk of the treatment - remember to wake them up at the end with some invigorating Tapotement so they return to their desk revitalised and ready for action!!

*   are unable to climb on to a massage couch for health or age reasons; this will include some people falling into the following categories -the frail, the infirm, some disabled and in the latter stages of pregnancy.

What are the contraindications to Seated Upper Body massage?

Contraindications are any factors which mitigate against the application of massage. These are similar to other types of massage. Each client's situation should be considered individually and even with each client his/ her situation may change with each treatment.

The following conditions should be considered by a therapist and a treatment may be refused or modified to take into account the current situation;
*   broken bones or fractures (unaffected parts of the body can be treated)

*   hip or shoulder replacement surgery or metal plates inserted in the upper body

*   any recent serious injury such as concussion to the head or a whiplash injury to the neck

*   cancer (to local areas and the skin) - ask about treatment requirements

*   excessively high or low blood pressure (check on medication)

*   diabetes, if the skin is thin as bruising may occur and there may be peripheral damage (neuropathy) to the fingers

*   drunk or under the strong influence of drugs (recreational or otherwise) - there is the risk that the client may become nauseous (caused by increased blood flow to the head) and may choke on vomit or turn violent/ aggressive or damage the therapist's equipment

*   high temperature or fever

* serious contagious skin and scalp infections such as impetigo, scabies (a skin infestation caused by a mite), conjunctivitis (eye infection caused by bacteria), folliculitis (infectious inflammation of a hair follicle), pediculosis capitis (head lice) and tinea capitis (scalp ringworm)

* minor contagious illness such as warts or cold sores (avoid the affected area)

* acute infectious diseases which are highly contagious such as mumps, measles, tuberculosis and chicken pox

* colds and influenza - the client will feel very uncomfortable if there is coughing and sneezing and these symptoms may be worsened by having the face in the face cradle; there is a risk of cross infection on the equipment and the therapist is in danger of catching the cold or flu

* infectious skin conditions such as impetigo (caused by bacteria entering the skin)

* serious muscle conditions or spasm

* prone to bruise easily

* bruising and unexplained lumps and bumps

* severe acne

* recent surgery on neck, face or other area (allow 2-6 months recovery time) and recent injections

* thrombosis (a blood clot within a vein)

* unexplained headaches and also migraines

* procedures such as Botox in the previous three weeks

* <u>pregnancy - no massage in the first three months (trimester) or if there is a history of miscarriage or other complications</u>

* sunburnt, inflamed, hypersensitive or broken skin

* eczema or psoriasis if it is in an 'active' phase when massage movements through clothing will probably be uncomfortable - balance this with the relaxing effects of massage

* diarrhoea and vomiting; the client will be worried about being 'caught short' and will probably not enjoy the treatment

* youngsters under sixteen years of age unless there is a responsible adult in close attendance such as a parent, guardian or appointed sports coach

* anyone the therapist does not want to treat for any reason e.g. a client has dirty clothing or deficient personal hygiene or has become aggressive or refused to pay/ turn up with no good reason in the past.

The therapist has also to take care if the client has any of the following;

* contact lenses, a hearing aid, a hair piece, hair extensions, a recent fake tan or expensive hairstyle or false nails

* balance problems for example as connected with vertigo or Ménière's Syndrome (do not rotate the head)

* epilepsy (do not rotate the head) and is it medically under control?

* thread veins or large pimples

*   moles (the client should be asked about these to exclude the possibility of skin cancer) and other skin blemishes

*   has an arthritic or joint condition which may preclude or need modifying to some finger massage techniques or movement of the neck, arms or shoulders

*   eaten a heavy meal a short time before the massage or conversely has not eaten a meal for a long period before the massage (take care when the client raises the head up from the face support cradle) in case blood sugar levels are low (hypoglycaemia) and there may be a fainting attack

*   cysts (an abnormal usually harmless swelling) or warts (a harmless although irritating growth on the skin).

A therapist should not carry out a treatment if he/ she is feeling unwell especially if suffering from a contagious condition such as a cold or influenza or has sustained either an acute injury or chronic condition. Serious thought should be given if the therapist is in the first three months of pregnancy.

The treatment consultation form

Seated Upper Body massage therapists should always ask their clients to complete a written consultation form which will alert them of any health issues which need to be fully discussed before a treatment commences.

The information given on the form and in conversation with the therapist will remain confidential and must not be divulged to a third party (such as a company who may be paying for the client's treatment) without the client's written permission.

The consultation form is a normal part of any therapy and the blank reverse side can be used by the therapist to write any ongoing notes about the client either before or after the treatment.

If there are any serious health issues arising which cause the therapist to doubt whether a treatment should be given the client should be asked to obtain written permission from their General Practitioner (Doctor/ GP) or specialist.

A supply of blank consultation forms could be sent to the liaison person at a company before a first session at a location. The staff members can each bring a completed form with them and this will save some time at the start of the separate sessions - the client will want as much time being spent on the treatment rather than the paperwork.

If a session is being carried out not in a fixed workplace and members of the public, e.g. visitors to an exhibition stand, are simply wandering in for a treatment the form should still be used but the therapist could guide the respondent through the form in a comprehensive but brisk manner.

The benefits of this type of massage

Seated Upper Body massage has many aims and these include - Improving concentration and alertness; relaxing tight and sore muscles; Improving the lymphatic and blood systems; helping relaxation and the emotions; decreasing blood pressure and eliminating toxins.

It should be considered a holistic treatment for the mind, body and spirit.

CLIENT INFORMATION
PRIVATE AND CONFIDENTIAL

Name ....Date of birth ....

Address...

Occupation...

Hobbies...

Home tel No..Work Tel No...............................

In order to get the greatest benefit from your treatment, please read the following information carefully.

BEFORE THE TREATMENT

Please tick any of the following that apply to you and discuss them with the practitioner. Please tell them if you are under the care of a Doctor or any other practitioner or are taking any prescribed medications.

Back injury	Stiff Neck	Recent Surgery
Neck injury	Back Pain	High or Low blood pressure
Shoulder injury	Shoulder Pain	Poor Circulation
Fracture	Numbness/Tingling	Arthritis
Osteoporosis	TB	Epilepsy
Diabetes	Skin Condition	Inflammation
Headaches/ migraines	Dislocation	Muscle Cramps
Bruise easily	First 12 weeks of pregnancy	Digestive Problems

Other...

Are you under the care of a Doctor or other practitioner?...

Are you taking any prescribed medicines? ....

....

"   Are you pregnant or trying to conceive? ....

"   Do you smoke ....Drink..................... (Indicate amount)...........

Please do not have a large meal in the hour preceding treatment.

PLEASE SIGN AND DATE THE FOLLOWING;

I have read the above information and discussed it where necessary with my practitioner. I take responsibility for alerting my practitioner to any physical conditions which may affect the work.

Signed...

Date..

What equipment is needed for a Seated Upper Body massage?

The following equipment is used by the therapist when carrying out Seated Upper Body massage sessions (some e.g. a clock, table and chairs may already be in the treatment room so it is good for the therapist to inspect the proposed room prior to working in it);

1. Ergonomic massage chair/ desktop massage unit/ kneeler chair
2. Low collapsible stool
3. Table and 2 chairs (usually supplied)
4. Receptacle for client's valuables
5. Client consultation forms
6. Client bookings sheets
7. Couch roll
8. Scissors
9. Supply of disposable face cradle covers; either gauze 'nurses caps' or soft paper
10. Baby wipes
11. Tissues
12. Antibacterial alcohol hand gel
13. (Massage chair) wedge shaped sternum support pad
14. Small towel
15. Clip or band for long hair
16. Small mirror
17. 'Blue tack' for temporarily attaching notices to walls
18. Clock or watch for timekeeping
19. Do not disturb sign
20. Notebook and pen/ pencil
21. Change (notes and coins)
22. 'Bongers' or other Hand held massage tools (electrical or non- electrical)
23. Mobile phone
24. Water and lunch for therapist
25. Water and plastic cups for clients
26. Therapist's brochures and business cards
27. Spare clean shirt in case the one being worn becomes sweaty or anything is spilt on it.
28. Length of carpet or an exercise mat to soften a hard surface
29. Copy of Insurance cover and qualifications.

Note: there is no massage medium listed above because if it is used there is a risk of a client's clothing being stained. This form of massage is done with the client wearing clothing and by not having cream or oil available; this will minimise embarrassing questions by the client about the removal of clothing. Music would be a distraction to those in surrounding areas so it too is not included in the list above.

1. Massage chair/ Desktop massage unit/ kneeler chair

The client has to be comfortably seated with the chest supported either on an ergonomically designed massage chair or on a desktop massage unit which is resting on the top of a firm table top. If a desk top unit is being used it is better for the table to be either resting against a wall or against another table; this will prevent the table moving away when the therapist is pressing against the client's back.

The massage chair which supports the client's weight should preferably be all metal (to prevent warping or fracture of any wood) and be able to support a client of up to 25 stones in weight. The chair should be well padded to protect the client's chest and be able to be well adjusted for different body shapes and sizes. There are any number of suppliers who have websites and who demonstrate their equipment at therapy exhibitions where they often offer discounts to prospective customers.

The problem with purchasing off the internet is that if there are any faults with the chair such as loose or torn fittings it may be difficult or expensive to return - always ask what the guarantee covers and are there any facilities for returning it if the chair is faulty. Also at exhibitions there are stands where members of the public are able to have 'taster sessions'. It can be instructive to ask the therapists doing the sessions what they think of the chairs they use.

Second hand chairs are sometimes offered for sale in therapy magazines; the problem with this type of sale is that delivery costs usually have to be added to the cost of the chair because the vendor is in Scotland and the buyer is in Plymouth!

The cost of a new massage chairs varies from under £100 to over £600 and with a more expensive chair you normally get more sitting position adjustments and better materials with more comfort for the client. Whichever chair is purchased there should be a protective carrying cover, sometimes with wheels for greater ease of manoeuvrability. The weight of a massage chair is about 8-10 kgs compared with 15-20 kgs for a portable massage couch.

A desk top massage unit, whilst it does not support the whole of the client's bodyweight is able to allow the seated massage to be carried out quite satisfactorily as the client's chest, arms, face and neck are wholly supported. The advantage for a therapist is that it only weighs (with carry bag) 4 kgs, can be carried over the shoulder like a satchel so allowing the therapist to board a bus or train easily, takes up little space at home and only costs up to £150.

A therapist when making a purchase should consider the outlay on equipment and calculate that if no work is forthcoming, for whatever reason, how much investment has been lost (this principle also relates to the cost of training to become qualified for insurance purposes). If a chair is purchased, it can be used for other therapies such as Indian Head massage, reflexology and ear candling as well as for Seated Upper Body massage.

Another cheap option is for the therapist to use an office kneel 'V' chair (with castors removed). This type of chair which is designed to promote good posture and back care in the office can cost up to £250 but there are some available at about £100 in high street superstore and office supplies catalogues. If this type of chair is used there will have to be separate padding for the client's chest and the face has to be supported by a small pillow or cushion which to many clients would not look as professional as a massage chair or desk top massage unit.

2. Low lightweight collapsible stool

A backless lightweight stool is important for the client to sit on when a desk top massage unit is being used as this allows the therapist access to the lower back. With a desk top being used the therapist can use a chair to sit on when working on the lower back, arms and hands.

If a massage chair is being used, the availability of a stool would allow the therapist to sit down behind the client when carrying out massage to the lower back and to the side of the client when working on the arms or hands.

It would be easy to carry and its use should enable the therapist to be less tired during a session which could last up to eight hours (with breaks). The cost of a stool is about £10 - £20 and they can be sourced from local hardware stores or therapy catalogues. If the stool has a washable seat cover this would be an advantage.

3. Table and two chairs

These items would be already available at the massage venue. They would be used for paperwork, for placing the valuables receptacle and other items. One of the chairs could be used by the therapist to sit on when carrying out the lower back, arms and hands massage sequences.

4. Receptacle for the client's valuables

The client's valuables - wallet, keys, mobile phone, glasses etc can be kept safely in one place (receptacle) and returned to him when he is due to leave the massage site. It is necessary for the therapist to keep the receptacle in eye view all the time so there is no risk of anything being stolen; by doing this the client will be reassured and more relaxed.

5. Client consultation forms

We have already discussed in this chapter the importance of this form which indicates any health issues which have to be discussed between therapist and client. These forms should be kept safely and the information on them not divulged to anyone. It is preferable if the clients can complete them before turning up for the treatment as this will save much time. The therapist should always have some spare forms in case an unexpected new client should appear.

6. Client booking form

The client booking form lists the daily attendance of those clients attending for treatments. Because the therapist will not know who is coming on the first day of treating clients at a location it is important for the therapist's liaison person in the company to complete the form and give it to the therapist before the start of the daily session of treatments. The form will have the company's contact details and also the details of the individuals to be treated. After the first day it should be decided whether the liaison person, who probably works in Personnel, HR (Human Resources) or Health and Safety, or the therapist will complete the form for the next time. It is more practicable for the liaison person to do this (unless the clients are paying for themselves instead of the company paying for them).

7. Couch roll

Couch roll has many uses and the main ones are;
*   to be used to cover up any internal windows into the room where the seated massage is being carried out; this will ensure privacy by deterring prying eyes (which couldn't see much anyway as the client is fully clothed and his/ her face is hidden in a face cradle)
*   to be used to wipe up any spills and to dry equipment which has been cleaned if the therapist has forgotten a towel to do this
*   to be a substitute for tissues if these have been forgotten by the therapist.

8. Scissors

The main use of scissors are to cut a slit in the face cradle massage gauze ('nurses caps') or paper face cradle covers which should be changed for each client. Scissors can also cut a therapist's 'snaggy' finger nail if one develops during a daily session.

9. Disposable protective face cradle covers

The face cradle on either a massage chair or desk top massage unit should be covered with a disposable face cover made either of gauze ('nurse's caps') or soft paper. A slit needs to be cut in the cover to allow the client to breathe easily The change should be made in front of each client and is important to;
*	stop cross infection on the face cover

*	protect the cover from being soiled by makeup

*	absorb any saliva dribble from satisfied (normally relaxed) customers!

10. Baby Wipes

Baby wipes are a convenient material with which to clean the massage chair or desk top unit between each client. This action will remove dirt, makeup and often sweat or perspiration from a previous client. The moisture of the wipes needs to be dried by using either a towel or couch roll.

11. Tissues

Tissues are useful for drying small areas and being used as a handkerchief by either the client or the therapist.

12. Antibacterial alcohol hand gel

Hand gel is a relatively new widespread introduction into the therapy world and conventional medicine, especially in hospitals. The aim of its use is to try to stem the problems of cross infection between patients and others. The gel is available without prescription from most chemists and pharmacies including those being set up in supermarkets.

The gel is an alternative and adjunct to properly washing and drying the hands. It is available in different sized bottles (250 and 500ml) and it is more economic to buy the larger size. Only a small blob of the gel is necessary and as it is very viscous it has to be rubbed into both hands very quickly otherwise it drips on to the floor. The therapist has to ensure that there is no allergy to prolonged use of the gel.

13. Sternum support pad

Made of firm foam and triangular shaped. Positioned horizontally it supports pregnant women; placed vertically it improves access to the shoulders and takes pressure off sensitive breasts. It can be used to support the neck during the head and face/scalp massage sequence.

MARKETING SEATED UPPER BODY MASSAGE

The Economic Background

Financial outgoings

Many complementary, including Seated Upper Body massage, therapists find it difficult to make a living from a sole source income derived from carrying out complementary therapies. Hopefully some of the advice and information included in this chapter will help increase net income and enable treatments to be carried out with more benefits accruing to both the therapist and the client.

Possibly the most important principle for therapists to follow is **the need for forward planning** to be made to maximise income and reduce costs. A simple example of forward planning which may be encountered is a request from a bank or other financial institution for a business plan to be provided in both the short and long term if financial assistance is being sought by an individual.

There are a number of costs which can be incurred to be taken into account and these can include;

* public liability insurance and any other insurances (essential)

* equipment costs including stationery, books and clothing (essential)

* income tax and national insurance contributions (probably inevitable)

* licence fees to the local authority

* membership fees and other costs involved with being a member of trade associations and other organisations

* petrol and other vehicle outgoings such as depreciation costs, membership of a breakdown service, servicing and the need for new items such as tyres and replacement parts

* telephone and computer expenses

* costs of training to keep skills and knowledge up to date [Continuing Professional Development (CPD)]

* accountancy and legal fees

* advertising in newspapers and magazines, the internet and on local radio and television

* property expenses e.g. renting and decorating a salon, extending existing buildings etc

* staff costs (if any are employed) including ongoing training, insurance and income tax payments.

Financial income

There are a number of sources of income which can be considered by a therapist and these include;

* treatment fees (work out the rate to give a reasonable return and check on competitors' fees)

* sale of products

* teaching and lecturing (obtain a recognised teaching qualification)

* writing books and DVDs

* writing articles for newspapers and magazines and appearing on television

* grants and loans from Government, and other, agencies (information can be obtained from banks, accountants, Business Link, Chamber of Commerce and government agencies and departments such as the Department of Trade)

* sponsorship

* working for an agency (check to see if you will have to train with them).

Marketing yourself as a Seated massage therapist

The following methods of marketing yourself are applicable to a therapist carrying out most types of therapy treatment. The therapist should be;
* **Professional in outlook and approach**
* **Be flexible**
* **Able to work under stressful conditions.**

Professionalism

The therapist should give the prospective and actual clients an all round holistic treatment and while the actual 'hands on' part of the treatment should be professionally carried out with skill and adaptability a client will probably appreciate the therapist observing punctuality and being sensibly dressed in a uniform which says something about the therapist. The appearance of the therapist should be clean, neat and tidy with nothing which could harm the client in any way. A therapist should consider wearing a business suit if going to meet a banker, financial adviser or company representatives if a 'sales pitch' is being made.

A therapist should make every effort to set a good health example to clients, certainly the therapist should not reek of tobacco smoke or alcohol and fitness levels should be reasonable. Many therapists do not realise how difficult bodywork is until they experience doing it for long spells during the day. By being fit the therapist is likely to avoid conditions or injury whether chronic or acute in nature.

It is very professional and impressive to the client that the therapist makes great show of cleaning and replacing any soiled equipment and cleaning hands between each treatment in front of the client.

If a therapist offers after-care advice to a client this supplements the actual treatment and indicates that the therapist has a caring approach and is multi-skilled.

The therapist's shirt or sweat top can be customised to display a logo, e.g. the author's corporate image - clothing, business 'strap line', stationery and books all have a common theme - 'Pressuredown Therapies'. When a therapist arrives for an assignment the clothing which is worn makes a statement of intent, this implies confidence and may generate enquiries from people in a location who may not be aware of the therapist's presence. The addition of a slogan on clothing is relatively cheap and can be carried out by specialists whose details can be found in a telephone directory or by the therapist if he/ she has access to a computer (there are many software programmes which can be used on a computer).

The stationery of a therapist says a lot about him/ her. The therapist's brochures, business cards and letterheads can be customised with colour, photographs or illustrations to make them more attractive and informative. The design and production can be done either by a printer, or the therapist using appropriate computer software. Remember that design costs are often in addition to the printing costs. Business cards can be supplied free of charge by companies, such as Vistaprint, whose details are to be found on the internet. Business cards should be given to clients and when they are on a massage chair left in a shoe so that it has to be handled by the client and not just stuffed in an obscure pocket or compartment in a handbag!

It is advisable for a therapist to obtain several quotations for any work to be carried out or any services which are to be provided. Looking at similar situations for other therapists and word of mouth recommendations are valuable. Often the cheapest quote is not the best value for money. Delivery charges, VAT and local taxes, and guarantee information should be sought from a supplier and taken into account when deciding to place an order. Ordering well ahead of time should reduce stressful situations arising e.g. copying should be ready well before a course is taught by a therapist tutor so that he/ she is not subject to shortcomings caused by a copier breakdown!

The equipment a Seated massage therapist uses should be safe, clean and built for the purpose it was intended for. The equipment needed for a treatment session has been listed in detail on page 105. The main decision the therapist has to make is whether to use an ergonomically designed adjustable massage chair which will support the client's body weight or to use a desk top massage unit where only the client's arms, chest and face/ neck are supported.

Therapists should reflect that the massage chair while having the main advantages that it will be able to support the whole of the client's bodyweight and looks impressive does have some major disadvantages compared to a desk top unit these are;

* more awkward to put away, carry and transport (it is not popular on crowded buses and train compartments)

* more bulky to store when not in use

* not as adaptable for use for many disabled and visually impaired people and those with certain medical conditions or who have serious knee problems

* normally a more expensive investment (a serious consideration if little work is generated for any reason)

* its appearance terrifies some nervous people - it reminds them of a dentist's treatment chair.

If the therapist wants to work on someone sitting at an adjustable desk top massage unit he/ she will need to have a low therapist's stool (cost approximately £10 - £20) available to allow the client's lower back to be treated.

Be flexible

A therapist should be flexible in outlook and this should be reflected in the ability to change working hours and the length of time taken over each treatment during a session. If qualified and insured the therapist can use a massage chair to carry out a different type of treatment - Indian Head Massage, Reflexology or even Ear Candling.

If a therapist is working at an exhibition or on a trade stand it may be necessary to change break and meal times to allow the maximum number of clients to be catered for.

Be able to work under stressful conditions

It is a great myth that every therapist is stress free because of knowledge which is possessed. The opposite situation is often very true and stress levels are raised when there are 'no show' clients or students on courses who do not come for any good reason.

A therapist should be able to rise above all obstacles and if he/ she meditates or feels 'grounded' this will help the therapist stay focussed on the task in hand. Good overall health and fitness will also help a seated massage therapist cope with working up to an eight hour treating day, possibly in a hot or dusty environment, although shortly after qualifying a shorter day of four to six hours will be more practical by being less tiring on the therapist.

THE TARGET MARKET

As we have seen, there are a number of locations where Seated Upper Body massage can be conducted and different groups who can be targeted by the therapist. In some cases therapists might like to employ the broad brush approach and endeavour to treat everyone. Other therapists on the other hand might want to specialise, possibly to tie in with an interest such as sports participation and contacts or because there is a feeling that a certain group such as the disabled might be amenable to the therapist's values.

The main categories of potential clients are;
* **Corporate market and production facilities**
* **Exhibitions, trade shows, product launches and conventions**
* **Sports events**
* **Department stores and shopping centres/ malls**
* **Music and other types of festivals**
* **Disabled people and groups.**

The Corporate market and production facilities

The main place to work in the corporate market is in the office. There should be enough members of staff to make the visit economic and the therapist can work either in a private area or at the workstation which would mean that the clients do not have to move away from their location. There are a number of 'white collar' sectors who use seated massage therapists, these include;
* **financial institutions including banks and insurance companies**
* **advertising, PR and the media (including TV, radio, film and photographic studios)**
* **publishing houses**
* **telephone call centres**
* **architects and surveyors**
* **legal profession**
* **dental practices, hair salons and spas**
* **emergency services such as the Fire and Rescue Service**

How to get into a corporate organisation?

There are a number of ways for a therapist to gain work in the corporate market and these include;

By reading the financial section of newspapers and specialist magazines and seeing which companies are doing well and are expanding their workforce make an application to this type of company by email or letter requesting to be invited to give a presentation, preferably including a couple of short 'taster' treatments. It is important for the therapist to make an initial written application (by letter or email) to the correct department [usually Human Resources (HR)] and if possible to a senior person who can take a decision. If no reply is received to the initial letter a follow up telephone call can be made. The therapist should send a copy of his/ her brochure and take along a copy of insurance cover and qualifications and a DVD showing a treatment taking place. An example of a specimen proposal letter to a company is shown on page 119.

Try to find out which companies have a good (or non-existent) stress management programme for their staff. Seated Upper Body Massage could be incorporated or introduced into the programme.

SPECIMEN SEATED MASSAGE COMPANY PROPOSAL LETTER

To be addressed to the Managing Director/ CEO/ Head of Human Resources by name, not simply title (obtained by a prior phone call to a company or organisation). If no reply is received to this initial letter a follow up phone call can be made by the therapist.

Date

Dear Mr/ Mrs   ,
Seated Upper Body Workplace Massage

I am writing to inform you about a form of treatment I am insured and qualified to carry out which you may find of great benefit to your company either in your offices and/ or production facility.

I have enclosed a copy of my brochure about Workplace Seated Massage which I hope you will take a few minutes to read and then pass on to the appropriate person in your company who can decide how it can be introduced to assist your staff and your company. It can complement other methods you are using to **help improve the finances and profitability of your company.**

Seated Workplace Massage is;
*   **Very cost effective when introduced into your company**
*   **A method to help promote and reinforce your company's image with the staff; helps reward good performance and reduces absenteeism**
*   **A method to help promote your company's image with the public and help attract new staff**
*   **A way of reducing possible work place health issues and litigation**
*   **Very quick to carry out - only up to 20 minutes per staff member**
*   **Needs little space to be carried out and it can even be done at the workstation**
*   **Done with no clothing being removed or oils being used.**

I would be very pleased to come and discuss with you or your other decision makers the benefits of this type of therapy which is being increasingly successfully introduced into all sectors of the economy. I will be able to demonstrate the therapy in action on several members of staff and explain how easy it is to implement.

I look forward to hearing from you shortly to arrange for an appointment to be made for me to visit your company.
Yours sincerely,

Name of therapist
Encl. Copy of brochure about Seated Upper Body Massage and business card

A company is likely to want to learn more about the therapist and if the therapist has a website this can be accessed by the company. The therapist should ask about parking facilities and request expenses (which could be defrayed against the first visit fees).

During the presentation the therapist could ask (i) when a decision would be taken about offering work, (ii) who will be paying the therapist - the client or the company, (iii) what are the company's procedures on paying fees, (iv) to see the room where the treatments will be given, (v) will there be parking facilities and the use of a canteen, (vi) what duration should each massage take. The therapist will be expected to say how much the company will be charged for each session; **the therapist shouldn't charge too low.**

Companies and other organisations often have in place schemes for monitoring value for money for their investments and these schemes often incorporate feedback forms which can be analysed to improve matters. A Specimen Client Feedback form is shown on page 121.

Payment for Treatments
Payment for treatments can be by:
* **The Company or organisation**
* **The client(s)**
* **A split between the company/client.**

It will be more convenient if the company pays for the treatments, any invoices submitted should have a time limit for payment ie 28 days. If you prepare the invoice in advance and hand it over on the treatment day it cannot be 'lost in the post'! Always keep a copy.

SPECIMEN SEATED MASSAGE CLIENT FEEDBACK FORM

To be completed by each client after a treatment. A supply of these forms can be given by the therapist to the liaison person at the company/ organisation who is using the therapist at the workplace or elsewhere. The completed forms should be given to the company representative by the client and the findings discussed with the therapist. The forms can be either completed anonymously or signed by the client.

Feedback forms are designed to show the firm that value for money is being achieved and also for strengths/ weaknesses of treatments to made known to the therapist (and any necessary actions to be taken).

Name.............................   Department..................................

Telephone number (extension)...................…….. Email...........................

Date of Seated Massage treatment.................
Name of therapist...................

1.   Were you given a consultation form to complete?   Yes..... No.....
2.   Did the therapist explain the treatment?   Yes..... No.......
3.   Did the therapist explain about the 'chair'/ unit?   Yes..... No.....
4.   Did the therapist ask how you felt during the session?   Yes..... No.....
5.   Did the therapist keep to the session deadline?   Yes.... No.....
6.   Did the therapist offer any post treatment advice?   Yes.... No.....
7.   Did you enjoy the treatment?   Yes..... No.....
8.   Would you benefit from another treatment? Yes..... No..... Don't know.....
9.   Have you benefited from past similar treatments?   Yes.....No......
10. Any further comments below would be greatly welcomed:

Thank you for completing this feedback form and its findings will be used to help maintain and improve the service offered to you. Any information transmitted to the therapist will be on a confidential basis and no names of feedback responders will be given to the therapist.

[Name of company representative]...................................... Date...............

* By finding out, and approaching, those companies that are suffering from absenteeism on certain days (Fridays and Mondays are most popular) or a fall in output due to stress related conditions or other conditions such as back problems or RSI (the company will never admit that it is work which is causing the problem for litigation reasons)

By meeting, and talking to, people from companies at business networking meetings and persuading them of the advantages to be gained from trying Seated massage in their companies - cutting absenteeism, reducing the need for expensive temps and agency workers to cover staff who are away from work because of stress and work related conditions and improving their image when retaining existing staff or recruiting new staff there is a possibility that the therapist will get work from this source. The therapist can stress that generally the introduction of Seated massage will save the company money.

There are a great number of local business clubs which meet regularly whose main aim is the referral of business leads between members and visitors and whose members learn firsthand about different professions and trades. Many have different rules and in the UK they include; Business Networking International (BNI), Independent Network Club (INC), Business to Business, Women in Rural Enterprise (WiRE) and 'The Business Club'. Details of the different business clubs can normally either be obtained from search engines like Google on the internet or from the local Chamber of Commerce or Business Link whose contact details can be obtained from a local library, local council offices or the internet. The clubs have different criteria for membership and membership fees - often a therapist can go as a visitor either through an invitation from an existing member or after contacting the Secretary of the club in question. It is a good idea for a therapist to visit and compare several different clubs to see which one is most suitable. Therapists can also make contacts in the corporate world by visiting and being invited to talk (often with a small fee) to local branches of national groups in the UK such the Women's Institute (WI), Townswomen's Guild (TG), National Farmers Union, Lions, Rotary etc The details of these local groups can often be found in a local newspaper which carries news of their activities.

* Often an invitation to give a presentation will come about by a chance encounter on a social basis between a therapist and the 'right' person at a company - possibly after a game of tennis or while sharing a spa pool when the company secretary complains of a bad back and the therapist can immediately say that Seated massage can be of help in the office

* A therapist may impress a company when working for it, or another company, at a conference or trade show and this may lead to an invitation to come and work in the company's office

* Each year there is an initiative supported by the government's Health and Safety Executive (H &SE) to raise the awareness of the need to protect workers' backs and the acceptance and furtherance of safe working practices. A few years ago the author was invited to work at the Mars Foods complex in Slough, Buckinghamshire where he was given working space in which he treated staff both from the offices and the production line. Many of the production line workers had not had a massage treatment before and a quick Seated massage was a good introduction to body work for them. In 2005 the campaign run by the H&SE was called Backs! 2005; in 2006 it was called Better Backs Campaign. For more information about the campaign and how therapists can support, and be publicised on, it details can be found on the H&SE Musculoskeletal Disorders website: www.hse.gov.uk/msd/campaigns/youcould.htm

* There are regular exhibitions organised by magazines, news papers and employment associations such as the 'Times Crème de la Crème' section which are aimed at highly placed and responsible office staff. If Seated massage therapists visit these exhibitions it may lead to contact with people who could make decisions about introducing the therapy into the workplace (especially in offices)

* Individuals who have been volunteer 'case studies' when a therapist was training may be keen to continue treatments after the therapist qualifies on a professional basis as paying clients.

Exhibitions, Trade Shows, Product launches and Conventions

Exhibitions and Trade Shows

Most industries and leisure activities have trade shows and exhibitions on an annual basis, or sooner, at venues which range in the UK from large centres such as GMex, Manchester, Excel in London or the NEC in Birmingham to small local village halls or town halls. At these events the organisers hope to have a large number of visiting members of the public and also a number of trade stands which have to be manned while the event is in progress.

Therapists can not only investigate attending therapy trade shows but also any other trade shows which have the potential for business. To reduce expenses it may be best for the therapist to concentrate on a venue in the locality. The therapist can research what events are scheduled in the coming year from the owners of the venue or their websites.

A visit to several exhibitions may indicate which stands may be more sympathetic to having a therapist presence for the public and show staff. These companies can be approached directly with the advantages of Seated massage being explained to the Head Office or the company's show agents. The size and position of the stand are important factors. As stands can cost many thousands of pounds the use of a seated massage therapist at up to £500 per day is not going to be significant in the economics of companies. The therapist can target those companies who are either very successful or conversely do not have any visitors to their stands. Often busier stands with more potential customers use an attraction such as a caricaturist, free business card raffle with champagne as a prize or fortunetelling - why not have a Seated massage therapist as an attraction to 'soften up' potential clients?
The therapist might either want to be paid by the visitor or receive a flat fee from the company. The therapist should take the items needed for a treatment session as appropriate. It is important to have regular comfort breaks and drink plenty of water as the atmosphere at shows can be extremely dehydrating.

At a show or exhibition the therapist can make contacts with companies who might want to use the therapist in their offices or production facilities. A colleague of the Author made some useful contacts in the London publishing industry when he met them at the Frankfurt Book Fair!

Product launches

Very often a company might be able to include in its budget for a product launch the inclusion of Seated massage at the event. Products such as new models of cars or electronics are launched nationally, regionally and locally. If a new car is being publicised it may be useful to contact the local dealership to see if anything is being planned. It is probable that the dealership and not the members of the public will be paying the therapist and that 5 - 10 minute treatments will be requested. Often at these events alcohol is served so be careful not to treat anyone who has had more than one glass of wine (or equivalent). Some dealerships have more than one location so if feedback is good there may be opportunities for additional work.

Conventions

There are two main ways that Seated massage can be used at conventions and these are;
*   to relax the speakers before they address the delegates in the audience
*   to be used to treat the delegates when they have some spare time between seminars and sessions - it is a nice, healthy alternative to going to the bar!

Therapists can find out the schedule of forthcoming conventions by approaching large hotels and exhibition halls where they are held also university campuses which are used out of term time. Most major bodies such as the Institute of Directors, the British Medical Association and the numerous Chartered Institutes all have annual conventions with many delegates. Again local venues will cut down on therapists' travelling expenses.

Sports Events

Seated Upper Body massage is an ideal way of treating two groups of people who attend sports events. These are (a) the participants and (b) the spectators, participants' back up staff and the event organisers.

(a)   **The participants:** Seated massage because it can be quick and is able to be carried out in most sporting environments - in changing rooms, outside a horse collecting ring, by a golf driving range or putting area, on the rowing slipway, near a motor cycling pit lane etc is an ideal method of carrying out last minute bodywork. Some contestants such as archers, horse riders, bowlers or shooters may need relaxing and others such as rowers, sailors, racquets players, boxers or martial artists may need invigorating before their event. The needs of each receiver are different and the massage should be tailored to fit needs as necessary. Activities such as mountain climbing, cycling, motor cycling and racing, tug of war and painting as well as those shown above might lead to chronic hand and arm conditions which would benefit from the remedial aspects of Seated Upper Body massage.

While it is preferable for the treatment to be done in privacy because no clothing is removed (except boots or helmets) there is no need for the receivers to be shy (onlookers usually soon become bored looking at others receiving a treatment). If young people under 16 are being treated it is necessary for a responsible adult to be present at all times during the treatment. For all people a consultation form should be completed. During the treatment the therapist can offer advice but it should be remembered that the receiver may already be advised by a coach, trainer or medical practitioner. The lack of use of massage oil or cream will eliminate any risk of an intolerance reaction to this medium which is traditionally associated with massage and which could affect sports performance at the wrong time.

Seated Upper Body massage is especially good for many sportspeople with disabilities; especially those in wheelchairs or who are visually impaired who may experience difficulty climbing on to a massage couch even one with electric/ hydraulic lift. A desk top massage unit would be advantageous for those who are not able to sit in an ergonomic massage chair.

It should not be forgotten that massage is also good as a post event treatment in removing muscle waste and stretching tissues. The element of stretching in Seated massage plays an important part in the overall warm down massage. Many of the other massage movements used will be probably slow and long.

There are several ways that a Seated massage therapist can be accepted to work in the sporting arena (consider both able bodied and disabled);

* by arrangement with a sportsperson, team or club or agent

* by invitation from an event sponsor

* by arrangement with a sports governing body or national association

* by being part of a sports medical team.

(b) **Spectators, back up staff and organisers:** Many sports take place over a long span of time (up to 24 hours at the Le Mans endurance motor race) and there is a great opportunity to provide Seated massage during this period. A therapist should look at planned sports events which are published at the start of the calendar year and regularly updated on many sporting websites to see if there any events in the vicinity. An early approach (by letter, phone or email) should be made to the person responsible for organising the event and a follow-up sent if no response is received to an initial enquiry.

If Seated massage takes place, the therapist should take care when treating anyone if alcohol is available nearby. Preferably, the treatment should take place under cover in a private area; this will provide protection from rain and excessive sun. A covering on earth will protect the therapist and the chair from any mud; care should be exercised on soft ground. The therapist should strike up good relations with those around him/ her so that neighbours will keep an eye on the chair and any other equipment if the therapist has to leave the site for any reason.

Often event organisers and sponsors will use the presence of a Seated massage therapist in publicity for the event as they feel this adds prestige to the event. The organisers will often pay the therapist a flat rate for the day, the other possibility is that the public will pay for their treatments.

Sometimes events support a charity and if this is the case the therapist may want to donate part of the fee to the nominated cause. It is not out of order for the therapist to make this clear to the public when they pay for their treatment. In fact the client may pay a little extra for the treatment if they know the money is going to a good cause. If all the money is going to a charity the therapist could ask the charity to provide forms which could be completed by tax paying clients which will allow additional money to be recovered from the Inland Revenue.

Department Stores and Shopping Centres/ Malls

The expansion of shopping centres and malls in the last 30 years in both city centre and out of town locations together with the franchising of floor space in traditional department stores has seen a diversity of services offered to customers. As well as offering clothes, household goods and food etc there has been an expansion in services such as restaurants, multi - screen cinemas and complementary therapies like Seated massage.

Seated massage is an ideal therapy because the equipment needed takes up little space and no clothing is removed so protecting the client's modesty. Treatments offered range from 5 to 20 minutes and this short length of time is ideal for busy shoppers and often their tired partner or friend who may be accompanying them on their spending spree. Carrying heavy shopping bags can put a strain on the upper body and this can be eased by a comfortable treatment.

Most treatment areas are franchised out and the period has to be negotiated with the managing agents for the shopping centre. It is important for the therapist to ensure that the possessions of the client and him/ herself are in view at all times as the opportunities for theft to take place are much greater when there are a number of people passing by the massage chair. Very often unsocial times have to be covered with weekend opening hours being the norm nowadays. Peak times are bank holidays with Christmas being extra busy. If the floor is marble or hard stone the therapist should put down a covering such as a short roll of carpet to soften the surface and protect the therapist's calves.

Music and other types of festival

There has been a proliferation and growth of music and other types of cultural festivals in the UK and worldwide since the 1960s. Whilst music may be the main attraction for the audience there has grown up a number of other activities which have been attached to the main event. These activities include healthy living, ethnic foods, children's events, healing fields and complementary therapies.

Most festival organisers charge the therapists for their pitches and after that the therapist is entitled to take any monies which are paid by the clients. This is a much easier option for the organiser than taking a percentage of the takings. It is important for the therapist to book the pitch/ site as early as possible as space can be in great demand and often bookings are made for the following year. While normal hygiene standards must be maintained the therapist might like to dress more casually in a sympathetic way to the audience. Many therapists are employed by companies and take their own tents or camper vans to the festival site.

Protection from the elements is important to both the therapist and the clients. A balance has to be struck between working in a tent which may become hot and stuffy in a dry area and working outdoors, possibly in a temporary gazebo where more people can see the therapist at work.

Disabled people and groups

Many disabled people are unable to experience the benefits of complementary therapies not just because their condition precludes them but more importantly there is the difficulty of accessing facilities. While it is difficult for some disabled people to lie on a massage couch even though it has an electric or hydraulic lift the same difficulty often applies to the use of an adjustable ergonomic massage chair.

Many wheelchair users would have to move (possibly with assistance) from their chair on to the massage chair and its adjustment would then possibly be difficult to carry out. At the conclusion of the treatment they would have to move (possibly with assistance) from the chair back into the wheelchair - what a performance!

A much easier option would be for the therapist to set up a desk top massage unit; the wheelchair user glides up to the table and puts the face in the support cradle and places the arms on the rest. The face cradle can be adjusted and the treatment carried out. At its conclusion the wheelchair glides away from the table. If there are any problems with the wheelchair not being able to go under the table the therapist can carry out the upper back and subsequent part of the massage sequence with the client in a sitting up position. If a desk top unit is used then the question of the client sitting with bent knees is redundant.

Obviously, if a therapist is asked to treat a disabled client there must be a thorough assessment of the situation and each case must be treated on its merits. If there are any serious issues the client must be asked to provide written permission from the appropriate medical practitioner for the treatment to proceed. There are six million disabled people and those suffering with long term illness [source British Council of Disabled People (BCODP) website: www.bcodp.org.uk]. When you add in their carers and others who are not registered disabled this is a vast number. Many of these would be able to use either a massage chair or the desk top unit; others would be unable to use either piece of equipment.

It is estimated that there are 750,000 NHS wheelchair users in the UK (source; Wheelchair Users Group) and when you add the number of non-NHS wheelchair users the number is much greater. In Kent alone there are 35,000 wheelchair users out of 161,000 people with long term illness/ disability; the population of Kent is approximately 1.6 million.

One of the benefits of carrying out Seated massage on a mobile basis is that the premises being used should comply with the Disability Discrimination Acts of 1995 and 2005. By using a massage chair or desk top unit the therapist will be confident that the size of the equipment will be comparable to a wheel chair.

By offering an inclusive therapy which is potentially available to all, few disabled members of staff or sportspeople will feel excluded. This is an important factor especially if a wheel chair user is in charge of a company or authorises payment to the therapist!
If a disabled person has a positive experience with seated massage this will probably be conveyed to a carer and other similar disabled people in a club to which the person belongs.

A significant national organisation a therapist could approach is the Spinal Injuries Association (www.spinal.co.uk) whose motto is 'because life needn't stop when you're paralysed'. There are many local branches of national organisations that could be approached and their contact details can be found on the internet, at public libraries and council offices and in the local telephone directory.

STRETCHING and JAPANESE DO-IN EXERCISES

STRETCHING EXERCISES

As people become older their flexibility decreases and one of the most important areas of advice a Seated Upper Body massage therapist (and any other therapist for that matter) can give their clients is to follow a regular pattern of muscle stretching exercises to try to maintain or increase flexibility. It is important for therapists themselves to carry out stretching exercises both before and after a treatment session; this should help to reduce the risk of injury.

The rules of stretching

Please note that when performing body stretches;
* The stretch should synchronise with an out- breath
* The stretch should be held for a length of time e.g. a count of 6 to 10 (silently please!)
* Each stretch should take place on each side of the body to ensure body balance
* Each stretch should be repeated several times to educate the brain to remember the body movement and to maximise improvement
* As soon as a muscle stretch is felt no further movement is required - this should minimise the risk of injury during a stretching session
* The stretch should be passive and not ballistic (bouncing); ballistic movement is designed to mobilise a joint and not stretch a muscle - it should follow on from passive stretching
* Stretching movements should be done gently and smoothly, not fast and jerkily. If necessary if balance is poor the individual should hold on to some support such as an adjacent wall or piece of furniture
* Individuals have different amounts of flexibility from others and also within themselves. Improvements in flexibility through stretching will be gradual and should not be seen as being something which will bring instant results
* Stretching should occur during both the warming up and cooling down phases in exercise e.g. gardening or DIY or in a sports competition
* Certain stretches may be especially appropriate for certain activities e.g. calf exercises before and after ladder work, cycling or flying/ in a coach for a long period
* **If any pain or excessive discomfort is felt during stretching - STOP IMMEDIATELY.**

There are many different stretches available for each muscle group and specialised books are available on the subject; one good example is listed in the bibliography of this book. I have taught for many years the stretches which I have described in this chapter and they have been found to be safe if done correctly following the rules of stretching as listed above. It is at the discretion of others and their own responsibility if they wish to substitute or add other stretches into their programme.

THE LOWER LIMBS

The Calf muscles

These muscles extend from the back of the knee to the heel. The gastrocnemius muscle starts behind the knee and forms the bulk of the calf; under it is the soleus muscle which starts lower down from the back of the tibia (shin bone). The muscles unite to form the Achilles tendon (TA) which connects them to the knee. Contraction of the calf muscles pulls the heel up to produce a springing movement through the toes; this movement is important in walking, running, jumping and hopping

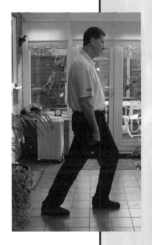

The stretching exercise
*   Place hands against the wall, shoulder width
        apart, arms to be held straight

*   Feet should be parallel and pointed toward the
        wall, one foot about two feet in front of the other

*   The front knee should be bent so that when looking
        down only the big toe is visible

*   The back leg should be kept straight and the heel
        of the back leg should be flat on the floor

*   When the front knee is flexed backwards
        and forwards a stretch will be felt in the back
        calf and this stretch will be held for a count of ten.

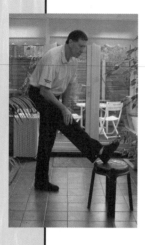

The Hamstring muscles

The hamstrings are a group of muscles (biceps femoris, semimembranosus and semitendinosus) at the back of the thigh; their upper ends are attached by tendons to the pelvis and their lower ends are attached by tendons, called hamstrings to the tibia and fibula bones. The hamstring muscles bend the knee and swing the leg backwards from the thigh.

The stretching exercise

*   Extend either leg so that it is straight and place the heel of that foot, with toes pointing vertical, securely on a comfortably raised support such as a chair, stair or low wall (note: the appropriate height of the support will be determined by the flexibility of the person stretching i.e. less flexibility = lower height of the support)

*   The other leg will be vertical with its foot parallel to the first foot

*   The weight of the trunk (upper body, above the waist) is gently bent forward until a stretch is felt in the hamstring of the upper leg (note: the stretch may be felt at different levels of the hamstrings depending on an individual's flexibility).

The Quadriceps muscle

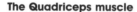

This is a muscle in four parts (rectus femoris (r.f.) and three vasti) at the front of the thigh with the r.f. originating from the ilium and the three vasti from the upper end of the femur bone. They pass over the knee to be inserted into the tibia by the patella tendon. The r.f. flexes the hip joint and together they act as a very strong extensor of the knee joint.

The stretching exercise

*   Stand upright on one leg and grasp the other leg by the ankle or bottom of the trouser leg (note: if balance is unsteady use a nearby wall, or similar, for support with the hand of the other free arm)

*   Try to keep both knees as close to each other as possible

*   Bring the ankle which is held up towards the bottom until a stretch is felt.

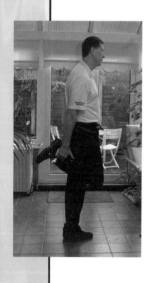

The Adductor muscles

This is a group of five muscles (gracilis, pectineus and Adductor brevis/ longus/ magnus/ minimus) which is found on the medial/ inner side of the thigh. They originate from the pubic bone and are inserted in the femur bone. They perform several actions including; adducting leg, rotating thigh, flexing knee and hip.

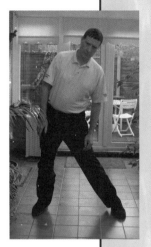

The stretching exercise
* Stand upright with feet slightly wider than shoulders width apart and parallel (FEET FACE FORWARD EVERYONE!!)

* Bend either knee until you can't see the foot on that side

* Bend the upper body towards the other side (the straight leg side) until a stretch is felt on the adductor muscles of the straight leg.

The Lower Back muscles

The lower back area is probably one of the most common to be inflexible in many people including therapists. The muscles involved are the Erector spinae and the deep spinal muscles which run along the spine and help to support it and the Quadratus lumbordum (which extends the lower back and side-bends the trunk).

The stretching exercise
* Breathe in and stand with both feet shoulder width apart, knees gently flexed/ bent and hands on hips

* Relax the body, breathe out and bend the trunk gently from the waist until the stretch is felt - do not try to touch the toes or stretch too far forward

* Breathe in and come upright and gently breathe out and bend backward from the waist looking at 'an imaginary magical golden bird which is flying over your head'

* Breathe in and return to the upright starting position.

The Side Trunk muscles

These are especially the external obliques muscle which rotates, flexes and side bends the trunk (upper body). Its origin is the lateral surface of the 5th - 12th ribs and the insertion is the abdominal aponeurosis (tough fibrous tissue which acts as a tendon) and the lowest three ribs. To a much lesser extent, the Internal and Transverse obliques and rectus abdominus muscles are affected.

The stretching exercises
1.
* Stand with the feet shoulder width apart (parallel and facing forward) with both arms bent at the elbow also facing forward with palms facing down

* Slowly rotate trunk in one direction until a stretch is felt and then rotate slowly to other side until the stretch is felt. Please remember to rotate the neck at the same time and in the same direction to minimise any strain on the neck.

2.
* Stand with the feet shoulder width apart and face forward

* Bend trunk to one side and at the same time lift arm on bent side up above the head until a stretch is felt

* Repeat the action on the other side until the stretch is felt.

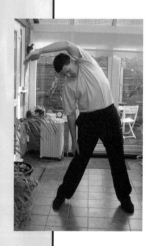

The Shoulder muscles

The shoulder is the area where the arm attaches to the trunk. Shoulder movements are made through two articulating structures; the shoulder girdle and the shoulder joint itself. The shoulder is a complicated part of the body and its mechanism is affected by many muscles which include;
* Trapezius; which stabilises the scapula (shoulder blade) and some elevation and rotation

* Levator scapula; which raises the scapula and rotates and side-bends the head

* Serratus anterior; draws scapula forward and rotates it

* Latissimus dorsi and Teres minor; adducts and inwardly rotates and extends the arm

* Rhomboid minor and major; which braces scapula and draws it down

* Rotator cuff muscles (Supraspinatus, Infraspinatus, Teres minor and Subscapularis); together have the action of abducting, outwardly and inwardly rotating the arm

* Subclavicular; draws the shoulder girdle forward and down

" Pectoral muscles (Pectoralis major and minor); together horizontally adducts/ flexes and inwardly rotates the arm and draws the scapula forward and down

* Deltoid; which has several actions - ant. = draws arm forward and inwardly rotates, lat. = adducts arm, post. = draws arm (extends) back and outwardly rotates

* Coracobrachialis; draws arm forward and inward.

The stretching exercises

Top of the shoulders

* Stand facing forward with feet shoulder width apart, arms hanging down by the side of the body

* Circle shoulders slowly; first in one direction and then in the other direction

* Raise shoulders and shrug them quickly, remember Bruce Forsythe (the entertainer).

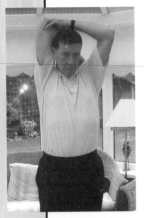

Outside of shoulders

*   Stand facing forward with feet shoulder width apart, arms hanging down by the side of the body

*   Raise right arm above the head and then bend elbow and place the right hand on the left shoulder

*   Then bring left hand to right elbow (which is still bent) and gently pull down on right elbow until the stretch is felt

*   Repeat the above actions on the other side.

Note: if shoulders are flexible it is possible to grasp opposite finger tips together behind the back. One side may be more flexible than the other. Take great care if a person is suffering with a chronic shoulder problem like 'frozen shoulder' or a traumatic neck 'whiplash' injury.

Front and back of shoulders

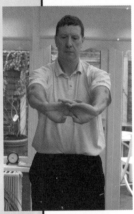

1.
*   Stand facing forward with feet shoulder width apart

*   Extend arms straight in front at shoulder level (if possible), with bent elbows, and interlock fingers so that the back of the arms hands face you

*   Extend arms fully; if flexible the arms should be held high, inflexible means that arms are lower

*   Return the arms to the bent position and repeat the action.

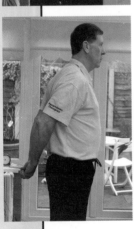

2.
*   Stand facing forward with feet shoulder width apart

*   Interlock fingers of both hands with palms upper behind the body

*   Straighten arms until the stretch is felt

*   Lower arms and repeat the action.

Note: It is important to ensure that the head does not nod forward during this stretch so that the shoulder muscles remain isolated and the stretch will have more benefit.

The neck

The neck is the part of the body that supports the head and acts as a passageway between the head/ brain and the trunk of the body. The upper seven, cervical spinal vertebrae are contained in the neck together with many important structure including the spinal cord, the larynx, the carotid arteries and the thyroid and parathyroid glands.

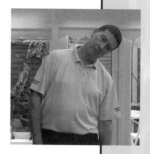

There is a complex group of neck muscles which are at the side and back of the head and all of them are involved in the rotation and extension of the head involved in the rotation and extension of the head;

* The posterior (back) neck muscles are the Splenius capitis and Sp. cervicis, the Semispinalis and Capitis which act to extend and rotate the neck

* The lateral and anterior (front) neck muscles are the Scalenes (ant., medius and post.) which side- bends and rotates the head and raises ribs on inspiration and the Sternocleidomastoid which flexes, rotates and side-bends the head.

The stretching exercises

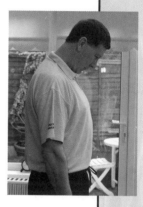

1.
* Stand with feet shoulder width apart, looking forward with hands on hips

* Gently lower the head towards either shoulder and stop when the stretch is felt

* Return the head to the centre and then lower the head towards the other shoulder

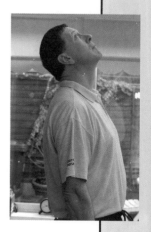

* Return the head to the centre and then repeat the action.

2.
* Stand with feet shoulder width apart, looking forward with hands on hips

* Gently lower the chin towards the chest and stop when the stretch is felt

* Return the head to the centre and then repeat the action.

The Forearm

The muscles and tendons of the forearm are important because if they become excessively stiff over a long period this can lead to the tendons becoming inflamed and cause the conditions commonly known as 'Tennis elbow' (lateral epicondylitis) on the radial side of the forearm and 'Golfer's elbow' on the medial side of the forearm. These terms are generic and the conditions can be caused by excessive repetitive use of a keyboard; it can be exacerbated by heavy lifting.

The muscles to be stretched are;

*   Radial (outer side of the forearm) - Brachioradialis, which flexes the forearm and the common extensors which extend and abducts/ adducts the wrist and hand

*   Palmar (inner side of the forearm) - Pronator teres and Pron. quadratus which pronate and flex the forearm and the common flexors which flex the wrist, fingers and thumb.

The stretching exercises

1. The radial/ outer forearm ('tennis elbow') side
"   Stand with feet a shoulder width apart, looking forward

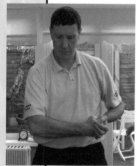

*   Bend right elbow to right angle, parallel to the body

*   Make a fist of the right hand and clasp it in the left hand
*   Press with the left hand until the tendon going to the elbow attachment is clearly seen (it is now being stretched)

*   Relax the hands and repeat the action with the opposite hand.

2. The palmar/ medial forearm ('golfers elbow') side
*   Stand with feet a shoulder width apart, looking forward

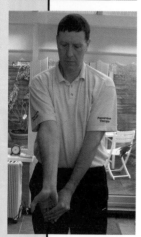

*   Extend the right arm straight and point towards the waist with the palm facing upwards and fingers extended

*   Press down on fingers of the right hand with the palm and fingers of the left hand until a stretch is felt in the forearm

*   Relax the hands and repeat the action with the opposite hand.

The Wrist, Hand, Fingers and thumb

The Wrist and Hand

*   Both wrists can be rotated in each direction several times and then waved about in a random pattern similar to that associated with an orchestra conductor.

*   The wrists should be flexed up and down through their full range of movement and at their nadir and apogee the position should be held for a few seconds. To achieve a slightly greater range of movement one hand can be pushed further upwards or downwards by the palm of the other hand

*   The hands should be independently parallel with the floor with the palms facing down, the hands should then be 'fanned' in both directions to the fullest extent

*   The right palm can rub all over the back and then the palm of the left hand; this movement can be repeated by the left palm on the right hand

*   The right hand can carry out Tapotement movements on both the back and the palm of the left hand - tapping, cupping, hacking etc; this movement can be repeated by the left hand working on the back and the palm of the right hand.

The Fingers and thumbs

The fingers and thumbs can become stiff due to repetitive action and pressure. To complete the overall stretching sequence they should be manipulated to relax them and improve circulation.

The stretching exercises

*   The fingers of the left hand can be rotated by the right hand; then the fingers of the right hand can be rotated by the left hand

*   The fingers of the left hand can be extended and then com pressed by the right hand; then the fingers of the right hand can be extended and then compressed by the left hand.

JAPANESE DO-IN EXERCISES

Japanese Do-In exercises are designed to increase physical energy and mental relaxation by stimulating all the major energy meridians. It is good for clients, who can try to incorporate these exercises into their daily routine, and for therapists on a regular basis, especially before they start to treat clients.

The sequence of movements can include;

1.   Stand with feet shoulder width apart and bend knees slightly
2.   Rub the palms and then the back of the hands
3.   Shake the hands and then clap them three times
4.   Rub along each finger, rotate fingers and then pull quickly on an out breath
5.   Raise the arms above the head and shake hands at ceiling
6.   Tap quickly and gently on top of head
7.   Brush quickly across the forehead with the fingers
8.   Rotate ears and pull ear lobes
9.   Rub up and down cheeks
10. Rub the side of the nose
11. Rub under the nose
12. Squeeze up along the jaw bone
13. Squeeze the back of the neck (good for relaxation)
14. Pound down the inside of the arm and up the outside of the arm (left arm, then right arm)
15. Hold the elbow and pound on the trapezius muscle
16. Pound the chest and scream out loudly!
17. Pound the back with the back of the hands
18. Pound the bottom with the fists
19. Pound down the outside of the leg and up the inside of the leg
20. Lift and shake one leg three times; repeat with the other leg
21. Close eyes and take three deep out breaths
22. Complete sequence by opening eyes.

Session Booking Form

SEATED MASSAGE

NAME OF
COMPANY..

ADDRESS...
....

CONTACT NAME ....
TEL:...................... E-MAIL...................................

Date	Time	Name	Treatment	Contact No.

SUGGESTED FURTHER READING AND VIEWING

Reading

'Anma: The Art of Japanese Massage' by Shogo Mochizuki
ISBN 1-57615-000-3. Published by Kotobuki Publications.

'Barefoot Shiatsu' by Shizuko Yamamoto
ISBN 0-87040-439-3. Published by Japan Publications, Inc.

'Indian Head Massage' by Narendra Mehta
ISBN 0-7225-3940-1, Published by Thorsons.

'Seated Acupressure Massage' by Patricia Abercromby and
Davina Thomson
ISBN 1-903333-01-6. Published by Corpus Publishing.

'Treat Your Own Back' by Robin McKenzie
ISBN 0-9597746-2-9. Published by Spinal Publications Ltd.

'Treat Your Own Neck' by Robin McKenzie
ISBN 0-473-00209-4. Published by Spinal Publications Ltd.

'The Complete Idiot's Guide to Healthy Stretching' by Chris
"Mr Stretch" Verna and Steve Hosid.
ISBN 0-02-862127-1. Published by Alpha Books.

Viewing

'Seated Upper Body Massage' dvd by Andrew Sceats
Available from Pressuredown Therapies. This dvd contains the
seated massage sequences described in this book.

INDEX

INDEX